G. G. Browning, MB, ChB, MD, FRCS(Edin), FRCS(Glas)
Senior Lecturer in Otorhinolaryngology, University of Glasgow

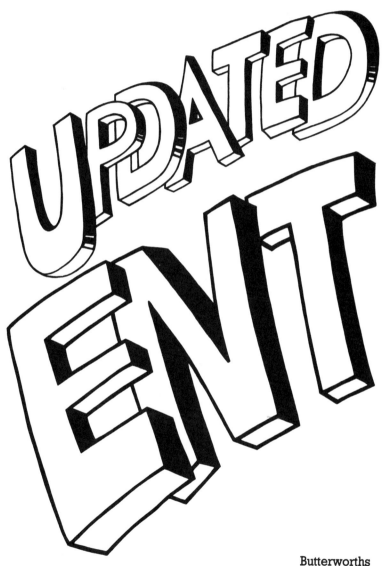

Butterworths
London Boston Durban Singapore Sydney Toronto Wellington

First published 1982
Second edition 1987

© Butterworth & Co. (Publishers) Ltd, 1987

British Library Cataloguing in Publication Data

Browning, G. G.
    Updated ENT.—2nd ed.
    1. Otolaryngology
    I. Title
    617'.51   RF46

    ISBN 0-407-00590-0

Library of Congress Cataloging-in-Publication Data

Browning, G. G.
    Updated ENT.

    Includes index.
    1. Otolaryngology. I. Title. [DNLM:
1. Otorhinolaryngologic Diseases. WV 100 B885u]
RF46.B885   1987   617'.51   87-11601

    ISBN 0-407-00590-0

Photoset by Butterworths Litho Preparation Department
Printed and bound in Great Britain by Anchor Brendon Ltd, Tiptree, Essex

Preface to the Second Edition

A text called *Updated ENT* requires to be brought up to date regularly and it is surprising what changes there have been in knowledge and clinical practice since the first edition in 1982. Thanks on this occasion are mainly due to Iain R. C. Swan, FRCS, for his helpful comments and for support as a colleague. Thanks are also due to the various owners and trustees of the following properties where, apart from my home and hospital, I have had the time to revise the book. Boston Museum of Fine Arts, Massachussets; Cleveland Museum, Ohio; Kansas City Airport, Kansas; Queen Elizabeth Hall, London; Tate Gallery, London.

Preface to the First Edition

The prime aim of medical education must be to train clinicians in the methods of arriving at a diagnosis so that the most appropriate management is applied. Many undergraduate textbooks do not take a practical approach, but simply list the various pathologies and describe their presenting signs, symptoms and management. They do not mirror bedside teaching where one is taught to elucidate a patient's symptoms and to give a number of potential diagnoses before clinical examination allows a diagnosis to be made. Students are mainly taught in Departments that slavishly investigate patients, often at great expense. This may be academically interesting, but students should be made aware that the majority of diagnoses can be made without any investigation whatsoever. Otorhinolaryngology is a specialty where it is possible to see the majority of the structures in which one is interested, although it can be difficult on occasions. Investigations are, therefore, perhaps less important that in other specialties. The main area that otolaryngologists cannot see is the inner ear and it is in this area that it is most difficult, even with investigations, to arrive at a diagnosis.

The aim of this book is, therefore, to instruct students in how to take a patient's otolaryngological symptoms, to arrive at a diagnosis by logical steps and then to manage the problem. When one takes a 'cook book' approach it is inevitable that one will be criticized. This is valid because there are as many different ways of arriving at a diagnosis as there are of baking a cake. Students should not be surprised if what they are told in their lectures and what they are taught in the clinics is rather different from what is written here. Indeed, they would not be receiving a University education if it were to be so. It is up to them to observe and, through practice and experience, to be in a position to be able to carry out their own recipes.

My education in English is abysmal and if the text is at all readable it is because various individuals have corrected the spelling and my wife has tried to teach me to express myself clearly. Finally, I thank all my numerous colleagues for their comments on these notes and for their support in running the University of Glasgow undergraduate course in Otolaryngology, for which this text was initially written.

Contents

The ear

The nose

The ear

Applied anatomy

The ear is divided functionally into three parts (*Figure 1.1*), the outer, the middle and the inner ear, and different otological diseases affect each part.

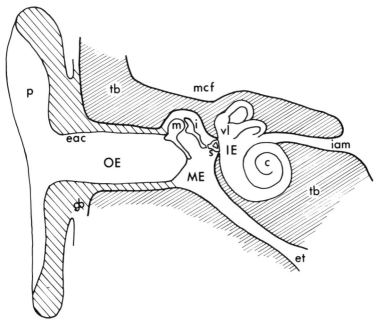

Figure 1.1 *Basic ear anatomy.* OE, outer ear; ME, middle ear; IE, inner ear; P, pinna; eac, external auditory canal; m, malleus; i, incus; s, stapes; vl, vestibular labyrinth; c, cochlea; tb, temporal bone; mcf, middle cranial fossa; iam, internal auditory meatus; et, Eustachian tube

Outer ear

The pinna (or external ear) and the external auditory canal are skin covered structures and, therefore, are mainly affected by skin diseases, dermatitis (otitis externa) and boils (furuncles) being the commonest.

The skin of the outer parts of the external auditory canal is different in that it has multiple specialized sebaceous glands which secrete cerumen. This partially evaporates, leaving a tacky residue of wax which coats the outer canal wall and prevents the build up of both foreign particles and normal desquamated skin by being shed. Wax retention may occur, especially where there is partial obstruction, for example by hairs, a twisty canal or osteomata, or where there is a surgically created mastoid cavity. Some individuals have a genetic predisposition to produce large quantities of wax but perhaps a more important factor leading to wax retention is attempts to clear out wax with proprietary cotton buds. This often does nothing but impact the wax further into the canal. The other culprit that will impact wax is the mould of a hearing aid. Since the resonant characteristics of the canal are not affected by the wax it is only if it becomes impacted that wax will cause a hearing impairment.

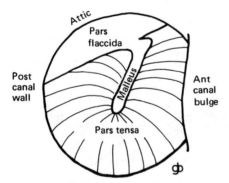

Figure 1.2   Anatomy of the right tympanic membrane

The audiological purpose of the external auditory canal is to collect sound and transmit it to the tympanic membrane, situated at the end of the canal. The tympanic membrane consists of a multilayered, fibrous membrane covered by a single layer of squamous epithelium. The fibrous layers are attached to the handle of the malleus, allowing sound to be transmitted to the inner ear via the ossicular chain. The main part of the tympanic membrane is called the pars tensa and the posterosuperior part is called the pars flaccida, above which is the attic (*Figure 1.2*). Middle ear infection can affect these parts singly or in combination.

Middle ear

This is an air filled space containing the ossicular chain. The middle ear communicates anterosuperiorly to the nasopharynx via the Eustachian tube, and posterosuperiorly to the mastoid air cells via the antrum (*Figure 1.3*).

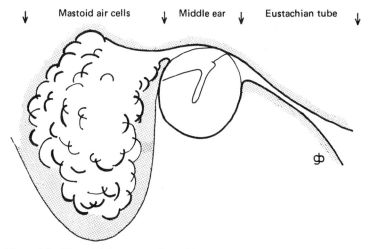

Figure 1.3   Air containing connections of the right middle ear

The middle ear and Eustachian tube are lined by a mucus-secreting ciliated epithelium. The air cells are lined by a simple layer of mucosa which, when inflammed, undergoes metaplasia and becomes mucus secreting. Serous otitis media is the name given to the condition when the middle ear is filled with non-infected mucus. Alternatively, the mucosa can become infected and the middle ear and mastoid air cells fill with pus – acute otitis media. Often the tympanic membrane temporarily ruptures to effect drainage. Chronic otitis media develops in some individuals when the tympanic membrane does not heal because of repeated infections.

The ossicular chain of the malleus, incus and stapes (*Figure 1.4*) transmits sound vibrations from the tympanic membrane to the fluid of the inner ear. The whole acts as a piston, the area of the tympanic membrane being considerably greater than that of the stapes footplate in the oval window. A conduction defect can occur in any part of the system. If the ossicular chain is disrupted, such as at the incudostapedial joint in chronic otitis media, a severe conductive defect occurs. If the tympanic membrane is perforated the hearing loss is proportional to the size of the defect.

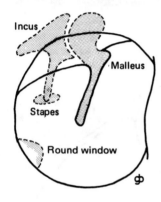

Figure 1.4   The right ossicular chain

The mastoid air cells are in close relationship to the dura and the middle and posterior cranial fossae. Meningitis and intracranial abscesses can, therefore, easily occur secondary to middle ear infection.

The facial nerve runs in a thin bony canal through the middle ear and mastoid before it exits via the stylomastoid foramen.

Inner ear

Functionally, this is divided into the cochlea and the vestibular labyrinth (*Figure 1.5*).

Cochlea

After arriving at the oval window, sound vibrations are transmitted in the perilymph compartments of the cochlea to the hair cells on

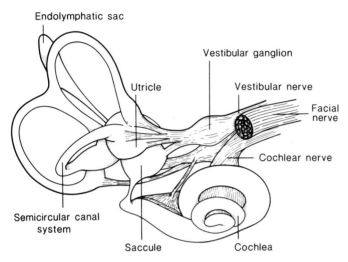

Figure 1.5   The vestibular system. This shows the relationship within the temporal bone of the endolymph containing vestibular system, its innervation by the vestibular nerve and the cochlea

the basilar membrane which winds up the bony spiral of the cochlea (*Figure 1.6a*). This allows sound frequency discrimination to occur. The high frequencies are at the base of the cochlea, and this is the region most commonly damaged in a sensorineural hearing impairment. From the hair cells, nerve impulses pass along the cochlear division of the VIII (auditory) cranial nerve (*Figure 1.6b*) which runs in the internal auditory canal along with its vestibular division and with the VII (facial) cranial nerve. It then joins the brain stem, interconnects with nerve fibres from the other side, and passes up to the higher cerebral centres. It is in the internal auditory canal that the VII nerve can be affected by an acoustic neuroma or a temporal bone fracture.

Vestibular labyrinth

The sense organs of balance are also within the temporal bone (*Figure 1.5*). The three semicircular canals record motion and the saccule and utricle record the position of the head. Neurological impulses from these organs travel in the vestibular division of the VIII nerve, along with the cochlear division, to the brain stem.

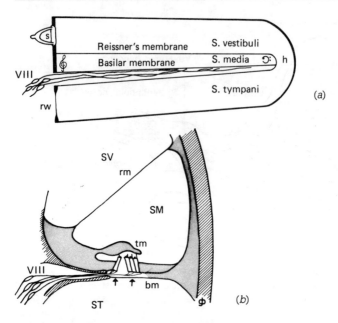

Figure 1.6 (a) *Schematic diagram of the inner ear showing the cochlea uncurled.* h, helicotrema; s, stapes; rw, round window; VIII, cochlear nerve. (b) *Section through the scala media showing the neural elements.* SM, scala media; SV, scala vestibuli; ST, scala tympani; rm, Reissner's membrane; bm, basilar membrane; tm, tectorial membrane; ↑, hair cells

Examination

The pinna and surrounding skin can be readily examined without the use of instruments but preferably in a good light. Operation scars are often difficult to detect because of their positioning in skin creases. Postauricular scars (*Figure 1.7*) usually indicate previous mastoid surgery and endaural scars (*Figure 1.8*) middle ear surgery, although any area can be approached through either incision. To examine the ear further requires a light to see by and a speculum to hold the external auditory canal open. Initially otologists used sunlight and silver aural speculae. The present generation uses reflected light from a head mirror, a power operated head light or a hand held battery powered auriscope with plastic or metal speculae. In addition an operating

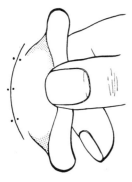

Figure 1.7   Postauricular scar

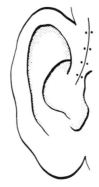

Figure 1.8   Endaural scar

microscope, which costs several thousand pounds, is frequently used in the clinic and is almost invariably present in the operating theatre. This allows the external auditory canal, tympanic membrane, attic and middle ear structures to be assessed with extreme accuracy. However, no matter what optical system is used, as large a speculum as the external auditory canal will take ought to be used. The pinna must be pulled posterosuperior before the speculum is inserted so that the cartilaginous bend of the external auditory canal is straightened.

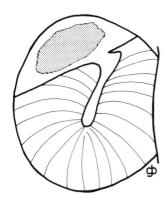

Figure 1.9   Most common site of cholesteatoma (right ear)

Beginners often find it difficult to identify the tympanic membrane, but if they are encouraged to identify first the handle of the malleus it should be easier. The attic area above the tympanic membrane should always be examined, particularly when there is an aural discharge, in order not to miss attic disease, especially a cholesteatoma (*Figure 1.9*).

A mastoid cavity in the posterosuperior canal wall is too often missed. Such a cavity is usually associated with a postauricular scar, and sometimes results from the surgical treatment of chronic otitis media where mastoid infection needs eradicating and the risk of intracranial infection needs reducing. How a cavity is created is best understood by comparing a diagram of the normal ear (*Figure 1.10*) with a diagram of a modified radical mastoidectomy (*Figure 1.11*).

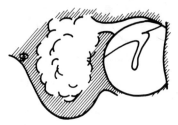 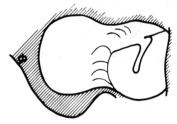

Figure 1.10   Normal anatomy (right ear)

Figure 1.11   Modified radical mastoidectomy created by removing the posterior canal wall

Every clinician should be able to examine the external auditory canal and tympanic membrane but it is usually left to otolaryngologists to examine the orifices of the Eustachian tube in the postnasal space with the aid of a mirror. On the other hand, there is no reason why every clinician should not be able to determine if the Eustachian tubes are functioning by assessing the mobility of the tympanic membrane.

This can be done by altering the middle ear pressure, either by the patient performing a Valsalva manoeuvre or, if he cannot do this, by the clinician using a Siegle's pneumatic otoscope.

The object of a Valsalva manoeuvre is to increase the pressure in the postnasal space, whence, if the Eustachian tube opens, it is transmitted to the middle ear, causing the tympanic membrane to move. The patient is therefore instructed to:

1. Take a deep breath.
2. Close off the nose by pinching it shut.
3. Shut the mouth.
4. Exhale, keeping the nose and mouth shut.
5. If the ears are normal the patient should then feel them 'pop'.
6. Children, and many adults, often find the above instructions difficult. They can usually be persuaded to blow up a balloon with their nostril with the same effect.

The clinician is, of course, looking at the tympanic membrane during this manoeuvre. If the tympanic membrane moves there is no need to do anything further. Failure of the tympanic membrane to move is most frequently due to the failure of the patient to relax his soft palate and, therefore, the Eustachian orifices are shut off. Get him to do it again and this time to swallow while trying to exhale against a closed mouth and nose.

If the procedure is performed correctly there are two pathologies that can be associated with an immobile tympanic membrane. The first is a small perforation that has been missed. The second is middle ear fluid. Because of the unreliability of patient performance, it is wise to try and move an immobile tympanic membrane actively with a Siegle's pneumatic otoscope. With such a system, the external auditory canal is hermetically closed off with the speculum, and the pressure in the canal is varied by pressing a small air bulb which is connected to the system.

Clinical tests of hearing

In an individual with a hearing impairment four aspects require evaluation.

1. **Severity of the impairment.** This is done clinically by free field speech testing, and audiometrically by pure tone audiometry.
2. **Type of impairment.** The impairment can be conductive, sensorineural or both. The distinction is primarily made by otoscopically detecting a conductive pathology or by pure tone audiometry. Tuning fork tests may sometimes be of help.
3. **Pathology causing the impairment.** Clinical examination of the ears will usually identify conductive pathologies, but tympanometry can be useful in the diagnosis of otitis media with effusion. The aetiological factors responsible for a sensorineural hearing impairment are usually suspected from the history.
4. **Disability caused by the impairment.** This is assessed by questioning the patient and by observing the patient in the clinic.

Free-field speech

To establish the threshold of hearing the patient is asked to repeat, as accurately as possible, words that are spoken to him. The point at which the patient repeats approximately half of the words correctly is the threshold.

Since there are two ears to be evaluated, it is necessary to mask the hearing in the non-test ear. One method of doing this is to occlude the external auditory canal by placing a finger on the tragus and then rubbing the tragus in a rotary manner. Alternatively, a clockwork noise box (Barany box) can be used but this is usually unnecessary unless there is a gross inequality in the hearing between ears, or if the hearing impairment is marked.

In order to assess the threshold of hearing there are two ways of varying the loudness of the voice. The first is the distance from the test ear: 6 inches is as close as one might wish to go, and 2 feet is as far away as one can stretch while masking the non-test ear. Second, the level of the voice can be varied from a whisper to a normal conversational level and then to a loud voice.

The words which the patient is asked to repeat should not be easy to guess; numbers like 99 or 44 are too easy. Either bisyllable words such as cowboy or hatrack or a combination of numbers and letters such as 9B5 or C3U are preferable.

After explaining to the patient to repeat as best he can the words that are said to him, the clinician stands behind rather than in front of him to obviate speech reading, masks one ear and starts off with a simple word so that the patient understands what is required. A normal individual in a quiet room should easily hear test words in a whispered voice at arm's length (2 feet). Indeed a normal hearing individual should hear a whisper at 18 feet but this is difficult to assess unless someone masks the other ear for the examiner. It is important to use a whisper and not just a quiet voice. In a whisper the vocal cords do not vibrate and the words are just mouthed. This

Table 1.1 Thresholds of hearing

Voice level	Distance	Impairment
Whisper	2 feet	Normal
	6 inches	Mild
Conversation	2 feet	Moderate
	6 inches	Moderate
Loud	2 feet	Severe

is most easily achieved by exhaling before whispering. If the patient cannot hear a whispered voice at arm's length, then he has a hearing impairment. Further testing will assess how severe it is. A whispered voice is tested at 6 inches, increasing to a normal voice at arm's length, then at 6 inches, and finally increasing to a loud voice at arm's length and then at 6 inches. The threshold of hearing is that distance and voice level at which the ear can hear at least 50 per cent of the test words (*Table 1.1*). The other ear is then tested in a similar manner.

Rinne tuning fork test

This tuning fork test may help to determine whether the hearing impairment has a conductive component to it. It does not help to determine whether there is a hearing impairment, this is achieved by free-field speech testing.

The basis of this test is that the normal ear hears sounds louder via the external auditory canal and middle ear (air conduction) rather than directly through the skull (bone conduction). However, if a defect occurs in any part of the conduction mechanism of the external canal or middle ear then the air conduction can appear quieter in comparison with the bone conduction. Thus, if the tympanic membrane is perforated or the ossicular chain disrupted then the bone conduction may appear louder than the air conduction (Rinne negative).

If the impairment is purely sensorineural then air conduction will still appear louder than bone conduction (Rinne positive). It is unfortunate that in many instances when there is a material conduction defect the air conduction will still be louder than the bone conduction. As such it is emphasized that the most reliable way to determine whether there is a conductive defect or not is to compare the bone conduction thresholds with the air conduction thresholds on pure tone audiometry (page 14).

Method

A tuning fork with a frequency of 512 Hz is normally used. This is activated either by pressing the prongs together or by lightly hitting them on the elbow.

The activated tuning fork is first held close to the external auditory meatus with the prongs in line with the canal and the patient is asked if he can hear the sound. The base of the fork is then transferred to the skull posterosuperior to the ear and the patient is asked if he can hear the sound and whether it is louder or quieter than when the fork was held at the external auditory meatus. If a patient cannot decide which is louder, the level of the sound from the fork, held at the external auditory meatus, is allowed to decay until the patient can no longer hear it. If the patient then hears the sound when the fork is placed on the skull, bone conduction is better than air conduction.

Interpretation

If the bone conduction is louder than the air conduction (Rinne negative) there is likely to be a conduction defect. If the air conduction is louder than the bone conduction, there may be no impairment (i.e. normal) or the impairment may be sensorineural, conductive or mixed (*Figure 1.12*).

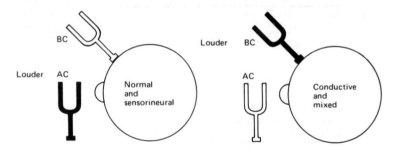

Figure 1.12   Rinne test

■ Conclusions

- The presence or absence of a hearing impairment is determined by free-field speech testing.
- If an individual cannot hear whispered words at arm's length then he has a hearing impairment.

- The severity of a hearing impairment can be graded by free-field speech testing at the distance and voice level at which words are repeated correctly.
- The Rinne tuning fork test may determine whether there is a conductive component to a hearing impairment.
- This is suggested if the bone conduction sounds louder than the air conduction.
- The most reliable way to determine whether an impairment is sensorineural, conductive or mixed is by pure tone audiometry, provided this is reliably performed with appropriate masking.

Audiometry

Audiometry can do several things more accurately than clinical tests of hearing. It can assess whether there is a hearing impairment and, if there is one, its severity and what proportion of it is due to a conduction defect as opposed to a sensorineural defect. On occasions it can also help to identify the aetiology of an impairment. Whether the results can be relied upon depends on several factors. Some relate to how and where the assessment was carried out and another relates to whether the patient was cooperative.

It might seem obvious that to assess the hearing the test has to take place in a sound-deadened room or booth so that extraneous noise will not affect the hearing but it is surprising how often tests are carried out in less than ideal circumstances. Another variable is the tester's ability to carry out the tests and, in particular, to use masking. Because sound readily goes round the skull and even more readily vibrates through it, masking the hearing in the non-test ear is essential. Suffice it to say that this can be difficult and if incorrectly performed will lead to errors.

The majority of tests rely upon the subject making a response such as whether he heard the sound or not. Such subjective tests depend upon the patient being able to comprehend what he has to do and then doing this to the best of his ability. When this is not the case, such as in infants or individuals exaggerating their hearing impairment to claim compensation, objective tests are required. The reason that objective tests are not used all the time is that they are not, unfortunately, as accurate as subjective tests.

Subjective tests

Pure tone audiometry

The patient is told to respond whenever he hears a sound. By lowering and raising the sound level at which pure tones of different frequencies are presented the thresholds of hearing can be assessed both by air and bone conduction. It is generally held that when the average air conduction thresholds are worse than 25 dB HL over the four speech frequencies (0.5, 1, 2 and 4 kHz) there is an impairment (*Figure 1.13*). If the air and bone conduction

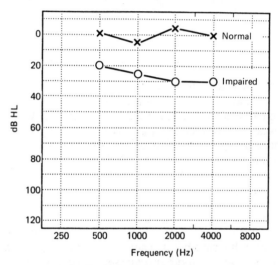

Figure 1.13   Normal air conduction (left x) and impaired air conduction (right o)

thresholds are similar the impairment is sensorineural (*Figure 1.14*). If the bone conduction thresholds are better than the air conduction thresholds, as evident by an air–bone gap of greater than 10 dB, there is a conductive defect (*Figure 1.15*).

Speech audiometry

The subject is asked to repeat back the words which are presented to him at various sound levels. This assesses the severity of the impairment and perhaps even more important assesses the subject's disability in understanding speech. There are many individuals with a mild, pure tone, sensorineural impairment who can never score 100 per cent of the words correct no matter how loud the volume is turned up.

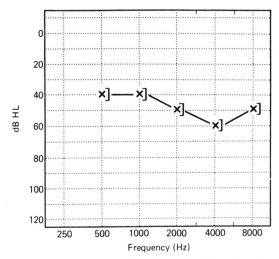

Figure 1.14   Sensorineural impairment (left) (left air conduction x, left bone conduction])

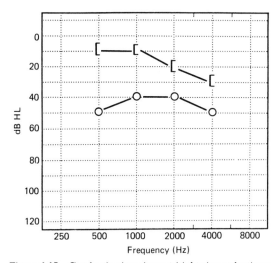

Figure 1.15   Conductive impairment (right air conduction o, right bone conduction [ )

Objective tests

Electric response audiometry

If repeated sound signals are presented to the ear, it is possible with electrodes and by computer averaging techniques to pick up the electrical responses to these in the cochlea (electrocochleography), in the brain stem (brain stem evoked responses) or in the cerebral cortex (slow vertex) and separate them out from other neurological, electrical activity. The thresholds of hearing can be assessed and, by analysing how quickly the responses arrive, it can be suggested where in the auditory pathway the pathology might be.

Impedance audiometry (tympanometry)

The test ear is sealed off with a probe which has three ports in it: one to change the pressure in the external auditory canal, another to introduce sound and another to a microphone which measures how much sound is absorbed. Most sound is absorbed when the external auditory canal pressure is the same as that in the middle ear. So by varying the pressure, graphs of compliance are

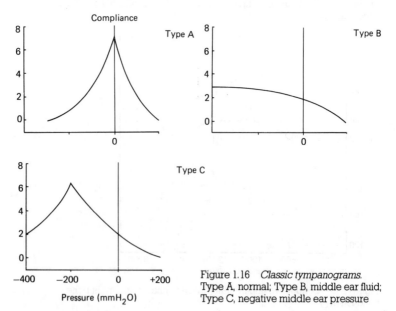

Figure 1.16 *Classic tympanograms.*
Type A, normal; Type B, middle ear fluid;
Type C, negative middle ear pressure

obtained whose peak indicates the middle ear pressure. A normal graph has its peak at $0\,mmH_2O$. Negative middle ear pressure is indicated by a shift of the peak to the negative side. Fluid in the middle ear is indicated by an a absent peak (*Figure 1.16*).

■ Conclusions

- Audiometry is more reliable than clinical methods in assessing the severity of an impairment and deciding whether it is conductive or sensorineural.
- Audiometry is not without its technical difficulties, the most important of which is the masking of the non-test ear.
- Pure tone audiometry is the standard method of assessing hearing thresholds.
- In those who cannot or will not respond accurately, electric response audiometry is an objective but less accurate alternative.
- The decision as to whether an impairment is conductive or sensorineural rests on a comparison of the air and bone conduction thresholds on a pure tone audiogram.
- Impedance audiometry may help diagnose negative middle ear pressure and otitis media with effusion.
- Electric response audiometry can help to determine where in the auditory pathway any pathology is present.

The commoner inflammatory pathologies

The nomenclature used to describe the commoner inflammatory conditions that affect the external auditory canal and middle ear is numerous, overlapping and confusing to the uninitiated. The conditions also present in different ways, so in this symptom-based text each will be included under several different headings. The following is an overview of each condition, with its synonyms, pathology, aetiology and symptomatology in order of frequency of the mode of presentation.

Otitis externa

Synonyms

Dermatitis/eczema of the external auditory canal.

Pathology

Non-specific inflammation of the skin and subcutaneous tissues of the canal causing oedema and increased epithelial desquamation.

Aetiology

Essentially unknown and likely to be a combination of the following:

• Decreased skin defence barrier.
• Trauma, e.g. from cotton bud, finger, match, etc.
• Climate/environment. Hot sweaty damp conditions.
• Allergy to poking instruments, e.g. nickel in pins.
• Bacteria colonizing an already inflamed epithelium.
• Iatrogenic. Secondary irritation to chemicals and eardrops. Secondary allergy to topical antibiotics. Fungal infection secondary to topical antibiotics.

Presenting symptomatology

• Ear discomfort/itch.
• Ear discharge.
• Mild hearing impairment.

Acute otitis media

Synonyms

Suppurative; purulent; bacterial otitis media.

Pathology

A bacterial infection of the middle ear and mastoid air system which occurs primarily in infants and young children. Spontaneous resolution usually occurs with rupture and drainage through the tympanic membrane. Rarely the drainage of pus from the mastoid air cells becomes blocked with the development of an abscess within the mastoid – mastoiditis. In addition, because of its proximity the infection can spread to the dura causing meningitis or brain abscess.

Aetiology

- Viral upper respiratory infections.
- Poor Eustachian tube function due to a combination of the age of the child and oedema secondary to the upper respiratory infection.
- Bacterial infection – usually with mixed, upper respiratory tract flora. Mainly streptococci, staphylococci, pneumococci and *Haemophilus influenzae*.
- Genetic/environment: commoner in the lower socio-economic groups.

Presenting symptomatology

- Otalgia.
- Aural discharge.
- Very rarely with the complications of meningitis, brain abscess or mastoiditis.

Otitis media with effusion

Synonyms

Serous otitis media, secretory otitis media, glue ear.

Pathology

Non-specific inflammation of the middle ear mucosa associated with non-draining of the resultant mucus down the Eustachian tube.

Aetiology

Unknown but likely to be a combination of the following:
- Poor Eustachian tube function.
- Adenoid hypertrophy.

- Recurrent upper respiratory tract infection.
- Repeated episodes of acute otitis media.
- Allergy.
- Genetic/environment: commoner in the lower socio-economic groups.

Presenting symptomatology

- Hearing impairment.
- Otalgia.

Chronic otitis media

Synonyms

Chronic suppurative otitis media.

Pathology

The primary pathology is chronic inflammation of the middle ear and mastoid air cell mucosa which results in permanent loss of at least part of the tympanic membrane giving a chronic perforation. There may be erosion of part of the ossicular chain, most commonly at the incudostapedial joint. Secondary hyalinization and sometimes ossification (tympanosclerosis) can occur in the remaining fibrous layers of the tympanic membrane and the suspensory ligaments of the ossicles giving an added conduction defect. The mastoid air cells become progressively obliterated by fibrosis and new bone growth.

A variant of this active disease is where there is in association a cholesteatoma which is a squamous epithelial-lined retraction pocket with a narrow neck which causes it to retain epithelial debris.

The course of chronic otitis media is variable. In some the activity is intermittent. In some it becomes burned out and inactive. Sometimes the vestibular labyrinth is involved giving vertigo. On a rare occasion, the disease causes a facial nerve palsy or spreads intracranially to cause meningitis or a brain abscess.

Aetiology

Unknown but thought to be a combination of:

- Previous acute otitis media.
- Previous otitis media with effusion.
- Poor Eustachian tube function.
- Recurrent upper respiratory infection including sinusitis and bronchitis.
- Bacterial infection.
- Genetic/environment: commoner in the lower socio-economic groups.

Presenting symptomatology

- Hearing impairment.
- Aural discharge.
- Vertigo.
- Rarely with the complications of facial palsy, meningitis or brain abscess.

Runny ears

As in many other medical conditions, for a patient with an aural discharge the history and clinical examination can be diagnostic. The main differential diagnosis is wax, otitis externa or active chronic otitis media. Acute otitis media is not included as its presenting symptom is otalgia rather than an aural discharge which only occurs in some. The following questions are usually helpful in deciding the most likely pathology.

What is the discharge like?

A discharging ear means different things to different patients and correspondingly the clinician must elicit its real nature. Some patients consider soft wax to be a discharge but obviously this is normal. However, contrary to industrial folklore, a mucopurulent discharge, readily identified by its foul smell, is not normal and is a sign of inflammation in either the external auditory canal (otitis externa) or in the middle ear (otitis media). On occasions, a mucopurulent discharge may be mixed with blood and this is most often due to the inflamed mucosa being traumatized by cleaning with a cotton bud.

Otitis externa and otitis media are distinct diseases and can usually be distinguished by the following question.

Is there an associated itch or discomfort?

If an itch or aural discomfort is present this is usually diagnostic of otitis externa (page 18). The itch makes the patient want to scratch or poke the ear and this type of discomfort can usually be distinguished from the other causes of otalgia (page 157).

Apart from otitis externa, the only other common cause for a discharging ear is chronic otitis media, where there is rarely otalgia because the chronic tympanic membrane perforation does not allow the pressure to build up.

These initial questions are usually all that are necessary to arrive at a diagnosis. Additional questions will help to assess the extent of the disease and dictate management, particularly in chronic otitis media.

What is the frequency of the discharge?

In chronic otitis media when the ear is discharging, the prime aim is to eradicate the inflammation. This will hopefully prevent the potentially fatal complications of meningitis and intracranial abscess. In some, medical management will fail and surgery will be required to eradicate the disease. If the discharge dries up there may be no further episodes of inflammation and the question is then whether surgery is required to improve the hearing. Other individuals will have recurrent episodes of inflammation and in these the tympanic membrane should be surgically repaired to prevent infections gaining access via the external auditory canal.

The natural history of previous episodes of discharge in chronic otitis media will, therefore, help in deciding management. However, it should be remembered that a high proportion of patients with an active ear do not complain of a discharge.

Is there an associated hearing impairment?

This question can be helpful in both diagnosis and management. In otitis externa, if there is any impairment at all, it will be mild. In contrast the hearing impairment associated with chronic otitis media is almost invariably noticed by the patient.

Is there vertigo?

This is an important question to ask if there is chronic otitis media, as a positive response would suggest a fistula of a semicircular canal. As this may lead to intracranial infection, surgery is usually indicated when vertigo is present.

Has the ear had previous surgery?

This question helps to avoid attributing abnormal clinical findings to destructive ear disease, as well as making the clinician pay particular attention to the posterior wall of the external auditory canal for a 'mastoid cavity'.

Other relevant questions may need to be asked but at this stage most clinicians would examine the ears.

How to examine the ear

Look for operation scars

Postauricular and endaural scars (*Figures 1.7, 1.8* and page 7) will be visible, endomeatal ones are not as they are deep within the canal.

Look at the external ear

Otitis externa often affects the auricular skin as well as that of the external auditory canal.

Press the tragus

In severe otitis externa pressure will cause discomfort, whereas in chronic otitis media it will not. Sometimes in chronic otitis media the bone overlying the semicircular canals is eroded. In these circumstances if the pressure in the external auditory canal is varied by intermittently pressing the tragus, the patient will experience vertigo because the semicircular canals have been stimulated. If vertigo occurs the patient is said to have a *positive fistula sign.*

Look in the external auditory canal

At this stage it is most likely that the discharge will be seen. Take a self-made cotton bud and cleanse the canal (*Figure 1.19,* page 27). Smell the discharge to see if it is purulent. Assiduous mopping should be performed until the entire external auditory canal and tympanic membrane can be seen. To do this efficiently, syringing (page 65) may be necessary. In this instance there is no need for concern regarding syringing an ear with a perforation as the ear is already infected. Once the ear has been cleaned the following should be done.

Look at the canal skin

In otitis externa the skin will be red and glazed and the canal will often be narrowed by oedema and fibrosis.

Look posterosuperiorly

To see if there is a mastoid cavity (*Figure 1.11,* page 8) and, if this is present, whether it is clean or full of debris and infected material. If full of debris, clean it out either by mopping, syringing or with suction.

Look at the tympanic membrane

The handle of the malleus is usually the easiest structure to recognize and from which to establish landmarks. Then assess whether the tympanic membrane is intact. If in doubt, use a pneumatic otoscope (page 9). If the tympanic membrane is intact it will be seen to move. If a rounded perforation of the pars tensa (*Figure 1.17*) is detected the diagnosis is chronic otitis media. In active chronic otitis media a perforation can usually be detected once the pus has been mopped away. Through the perforation it is often possible to see the inflamed middle ear mucosa. Sometimes granulation tissue or, more rarely, a polyp arising from the middle ear obscures the view.

In active chronic otitis media an alternative site of the disease is the attic, hence the importance of inspecting this area. The inflammation here is often associated with a retraction pocket of squamous epithelium which becomes full of debris (*Figure 1.18*). This type of chronic otitis media is called a cholesteatoma and the inflammation does not respond to medical treatment (*see below*).

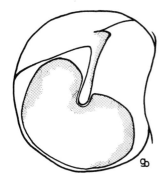

Figure 1.17   Right tympanic
membrane perforation

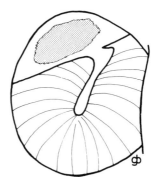

Figure 1.18   Right attic
cholesteatoma

In conclusion, if the ear is properly cleaned out it is usually possible, along with the history, to distinguish between otitis externa and chronic otitis media as the cause of a discharging ear. It is wise at this stage to test the hearing clinically by using voice testing (page 10).

Having made the diagnosis what do you do next?

As far as the basic management is concerned, it does not matter what the diagnosis is in a patient with a discharging ear. It is the same, aural toilet to remove the debris. Whether this is done by syringing or mopping with cotton buds does not matter provided it is done thoroughly.

The majority of patients with otitis externa or chronic otitis media will symptomatically respond to aural toilet alone. Many clinicians prefer a 'belt and braces' approach so the additional treatments that can be prescribed are discussed below.

Specific management of otitis externa

Aural toilet, plus if required:

1. *Topical ear preparation* to sooth and medicate. A large variety of preparations are available; 0.1 per cent steroid (betamethasone, dexamethasone) cream applied with cotton buds, glycerol and ichthamol or aluminium acetate ear drops. Antibiotics should not be included in any of these preparations as any organisms present are commensals or secondary invaders rather than the cause of the disease. Topical antibiotics often make the otitis externa worse by causing an allergic skin reaction or superinfection with bacteria and fungi.
2. *Wicks,* if the external auditory canal is too narrow. Impregnate a ½-inch ribbon gauze wick with one of the above ear preparations and change daily. This will allow the canal to open up and topical preparations on their own can then be substituted.
3. *Analgesics* if discomfort is not controlled with topical applications.
4. *Exclude allergens.* Enquire how the patient cleans out his ear and what he has been putting in it.

Specific management of active chronic otitis media

Following thorough aural toilet by a trained member of staff, the patient is told that he has to mop! mop! mop! the ear with a cotton bud. These should be hand made (*Figure 1.19*) as commercial buds are virtually useless, being both too large and too hard. Get the patients to mop, their wives/husbands/girlfriends/boyfriends to mop and the district nurse/hospital nurse to mop at least three times per day until the cotton buds come out dry. This is the only way to clean the ear, to allow it to drain and if any medications are being applied, to allow them to make contact. If thought necessary aural toilet can be followed by:

* *Topical antibiotic/steroid ear drops* four times daily for 4 weeks. These have to be instilled correctly with the head in a lateral position to ensure that they reach the middle ear. Topical antibiotics on their own are valueless as are systemic antibiotics.

The symptomatic response to such management is high because the ear no longer discharges as it is being mopped away.

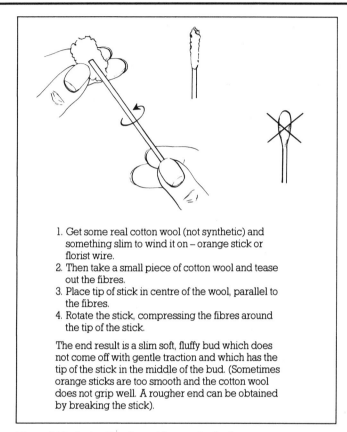

1. Get some real cotton wool (not synthetic) and something slim to wind it on – orange stick or florist wire.
2. Then take a small piece of cotton wool and tease out the fibres.
3. Place tip of stick in centre of the wool, parallel to the fibres.
4. Rotate the stick, compressing the fibres around the tip of the stick.

The end result is a slim soft, fluffy bud which does not come off with gentle traction and which has the tip of the stick in the middle of the bud. (Sometimes orange sticks are too smooth and the cotton wool does not grip well. A rougher end can be obtained by breaking the stick).

Figure 1.19   Instructions for making a cotton bud

However, the percentage of ears that become otoscopically inactive is not high and even then activity is likely to recur. Referral for specialist advice is recommended for all patients with an actively discharging ear due to chronic otitis media.

Specialist management of active chronic otitis media

The initial specialist management usually consists of even more thorough aural toilet under microscopic vision with suction and a course of medical therapy. If the ear becomes inactive serious consideration will be given to surgical repair of the tympanic membrane and any associated defects in the ossicular chain (tympanoplasty) with the double aim of restoring the hearing and preventing re-infection.

If medical treatment of the discharge fails, surgery will often be recommended to obviate the risk of meningitis or intracranial abscess. Surgery is usually a cortical or modified radical mastoidectomy, sometimes with a tympanoplasty to restore the hearing.

■ Conclusions

• Otitis externa and active chronic otitis media are the main causes of a discharging ear.
• The history of the type of discharge and the presence or absence of itch or pain are usually diagnostic .
• The ear will require thorough aural toilet before being examined.
• Clinical examination is also diagnostic.
• The essence of management of a discharging ear, whatever its cause, is aural toilet, usually by mopping or syringing.

Pain in the ear

It can be difficult to elucidate the cause of a painful ear, mainly because the pain can originate locally in the ear or temporomandibular joint, or it can be referred from elsewhere in the head and neck. Otological conditions are generally associated with other otological symptoms, most frequently a hearing impairment, and they can usually be identified by looking in and around the ear. Temporomandibular causes can almost always be identified by eliciting tenderness over the joint and on straining the jaw. If no otological or temporomandibular pathology is identified then it must be referred pain.

The diagnostic possibilities for otalgia are different in children and in adults, therefore they will be dealt with separately.

Otalgia in children

Perhaps the commonest type of history is from the parents of a young child, up to the age of about ten years. The child wakes in the middle of the night screaming and crying with earache. Usually there is a preceding cold or cough and the differential diagnosis is acute otitis media, otitis media with effusion, negative middle ear pressure or referred pain from the teeth, or the upper respiratory and alimentary tracts. To make a distinction is not easy but thankfully it does not matter too much. In all, the mainstay of management is analgesics such as paracetamol elixir.

Acute otitis media

Here the otalgia is due to a build up of pus under pressure within the middle ear. The diagnosis is made by finding a bulging, inflamed tympanic membrane. The mastoid should be palpated for tenderness which would suggest mastoiditis, though this complication is uncommon. This would have to be treated much more seriously to prevent the intracranial spread of infection.

The primary management is analgesics with the addition of antibiotics (ampicillin, amoxycillin) if the child is systemically unwell as evident by fever and/or lymphadenopathy. Antibiotic therapy is by no means mandatory, no major benefit having been demonstrated in controlled clinical trials. In most children, the pain settles rapidly due to spontaneous resolution or by rupture and drainage of the pus via the tympanic membrane. Some would prescribe nasal decongestants to encourage drainage down the Eustachian tube and some would suggest myringotomy. If mastoiditis is suspected, hospital management is necessary.

All children who have had acute otitis media should be reviewed to assess their hearing as a few will proceed to otitis media with effusion.

Negative middle ear pressure/early otitis media with effusion

In children this is perhaps a commoner cause of otalgia than acute otitis media but the majority of chidren with chronic middle ear effusion do not have otalgia. The reasons for this are as follows. Otalgia is only caused by sudden changes in the differential pressure across the tympanic membrane between the middle ear and the external auditory canal. So in the diagnostic situation being described the Eustachian tube is not functioning normally because of the oedema associated with the upper respiratory infection. The child is sleeping, mouth breathing and not swallowing, so the air is absorbed from the middle ear and a painful differential pressure develops.

The otoscopic detection of negative middle ear pressure is difficult at any time, and more so in a fretful child. Pneumatic otoscopy can be helpful. Crying should not be discouraged as it can help to get air back into the middle ear.

Teething

The referred pain from teething should be detected by eliciting tenderness over the, as yet, unerupted tooth.

Upper respiratory infection

Pain from the inflamed naso-, oro- and hypopharynx can be referred to the ear, further confounding the diagnostic dilemma. It is by excluding otological and teething problems that the diagnosis is made.

Otalgia in adults

Though the conditions that cause otalgia in children can also cause it in adults they are relatively infrequent compared with the following.

Otitis externa

The diagnosis should be evident by otoscopy and the management is as described elsewhere (page 26).

Boils

These can be acutely painful and sometimes difficult to distinguish from severe otitis externa. Local heat and analgesics are usually all that are necessary.

Negative middle ear pressure

The aetiology of this, as in children, can be an upper respiratory infection but frequently there is the added insult of changes in atmospheric pressure associated with air travel or diving.

Temporomandibular joint inflammation

This is almost always associated with major gaps in the dentition, loose dentures or non-wearing of dentures, which causes continued strain on the joint. The joint itself will be tender to palpation and pain will be caused by opening the jaw and shoving it to one side. The long-term management is by correcting problems of dentition. In the short term, anti-inflammatory analgesics are useful.

Cervical osteo-arthritis

Pain due to this can usually be elicited by rotating and or laterally positioning the head. X-rays are of minimum value as many older spines will be osteo-arthritic anyway. Management is with anti-inflammatory analgesics and perhaps neck rest with a cervical collar.

Pharyngeal tumours

Though uncommon in comparison with the other causes of otalgia in adults it is a diagnosis not to be missed. There may or may not be other symptoms expected to be associated with such tumours (page 115). Unfortunately, the presence of pain with such tumours usually indicates involvement of the glossopharyngeal nerve at the base of the skull and therefore a poor prognosis, however treated.

■ Conclusions

● Otalgia is as frequently non-otological (due to referred pain) as it is otological in origin.

- In children the commoner otological causes are acute otitis media, negative middle ear pressure and otitis media with effusion.
- In children the commoner non-otological causes are discomfort from the naso- and oropharynx associated with an upper respiratory tract infection or with teething.
- In adults, otitis externa, boils and negative middle ear pressure following air travel or diving are the main otological causes.
- In adults, temporomandibular and cervical joint problems are the common non-otological causes. A naso- or oropharyngeal neoplasm should be considered.
- Otological conditions are usually diagnosed by otoscopy. If none are present it is most likely referred pain and a cause for this should be looked for.

Hearing impairment in adults

In the region of 20 per cent of adults have a hearing impairment, the slightly higher proportion being sensorineural. The high prevalence of sensorineural impairments is mainly related to age, not that age itself is the cause, it is rather that the chances of being exposed to the factors that cause impairments increase with age. It is surprising how many older patients do not complain spontaneously of having hearing difficulties. This is probably due to a combination of the slowly progressive nature of most impairments and the expectation that the hearing will deteriorate with age. The clinician should, therefore, train himself to anticipate and identify hearing problems rather than waiting for patients to complain. Though patients often attribute their impairment to wax this is usually not the case. In older adults, sensorineural impairments are by far the commoner type, and although impacted wax can on occasions cause an impairment it is usually an additive, rather than the only, cause.

As sudden hearing losses present differently and are considered an otological emergency, they are considered elsewhere (page 51).

How to arrive at a diagnosis

A patient who complains of difficulty in hearing probably has! The elucidation of its cause requires a combination of a clinical history and examination. The history will identify any aetiological factors which might be responsible for a sensorineural impairment, the clinical examination will confirm the presence of an impairment, and perhaps elucidate whether it is sensorineural or conductive in nature. In the latter, the clinical examination will usually identify its aetiology. The history will also indicate the situations where the patient is disabled, which is important for management, as this is tailored to each patient. Pure tone audiometry is usually performed to confirm the severity and type of the impairment but the patient's disability is by no means directly related to the pure tone audiogram.

History

The order in which the following questions are asked will depend on how a patient responds, but answers to them all should be known at the end of the examination.

How much trouble is the patient having in hearing?

The disability that a patient has in hearing not only dictates the need for management but in many instances its form. It is necessary to ask the patient this question because disability is not directly related to the severity of the impairment as measured by voice testing or by an audiogram. This is for many reasons but not least the ability of the patient to overcome a disability by speech (lip) reading. Often the earliest evidence of an impairment is listening to conversation in a noisy background. With more severe impairments there will be difficulty in hearing in a 'one to one' conversation, listening to the television and using the telephone. Whether the patient has a particularly bad side should be noted as this indicates asymmetric hearing. It is not uncommon for a patient to attribute all his hearing difficulties to one ear, but because sound travels readily around the skull it is only in difficult listening conditions that a unilateral impairment will cause problems.

What is the natural history of the impairment?

Most impairments usually affect both ears and slowly progress over many years, but occasionally the impairment comes on suddenly. Hopefully, if this occurs, a patient will be referred to an otolaryngologist as soon as possible for investigation and management (page 51). Another type of impairment is one that fluctuates and, in the absence of other symptoms or obvious factors such as water, this is almost certainly due to otitis media with effusion.

Is one ear worse than the other?

The commonest reason why an individual might have a unilateral or asymmetric impairment is that there is a conductive defect in the poorer ear. To disregard this is not of great concern, but to disregard a unilateral or asymmetric sensorineural impairment can be dangerous because one of the causes of this is an acoustic neuroma.

Are they any associated symptoms?

It should be ascertained whether a patient has tinnitus, vertigo, otalgia or an aural discharge and, if present, further enquiries are as indicated elsewhere.

Are there any obvious aetiological factors?

Do the ears run? The presence of a smelly discharge, without pain or discomfort, suggests active chronic otitis media, but it is surprising how many patients with an ear full of pus state that the ear does not run.

Have they been exposed to noise?

Everyone today is exposed to unnecessary noise but this is usually of little consequence. The levels that should cause concern are those at work which make communication difficult, as exemplified by the need to shout. The risk of damage is related to the number of years of exposure but the risk can be virtually eliminated by the wearing of ear muffs or plugs. In any patient with an impairment his job history should be enquired about and a note also made about impact noise such as rivetting, machine stamping and shooting, as these produce a sensorineural impairment more readily than constant noise. Although disco music is loud enough to have an effect on hearing, most people are not exposed for a sufficient total number of hours for this to have a permanent effect.

How is their general health?

Many generalized diseases are thought to have an effect on hearing. The cochlea is supplied by an end artery and is likely to be subject to the effects of both peripheral and general vascular disease. Thus, a history of diabetes, strokes, transient ischaemic attacks, angina, myocardial infarction, hypertension and intermittent claudication would all support an ischaemic factor in the impairment.

What drugs are they on?

This follows on naturally from the previous question. Many drugs have been suggested to cause or aggravate an impairment, in particular, aspirin, beta-blockers and loop diuretics. Unfortunately, the only drug-induced impairment that is totally reversed by stopping the drug is aspirin.

The aminoglycosides are considerably more likely than anything else to cause an impairment but the mode of onset is sudden, is often associated with vertigo, and is usually clearly related to its prescription (page 53).

Clinical examination

By the time the history has been taken it will usually be fairly obvious whether communication with the patient is difficult or not. Inability to communicate should not be automatically ascribed to senility or idiocy. Although this is sometimes the case, it is surprising how much more alert a patient can become once he or she has been fitted with a hearing aid.

There is no set routine to the clinical examination but the experienced clinician will also have noted automatically, while taking the history, whether the patient is speech (lip) reading. The next thing to do is to test the hearing, especially if there is

TABLE 1.2. Simplified flow diagram of the means of arriving at a diagnosis of the cause of hearing loss by clinical examination

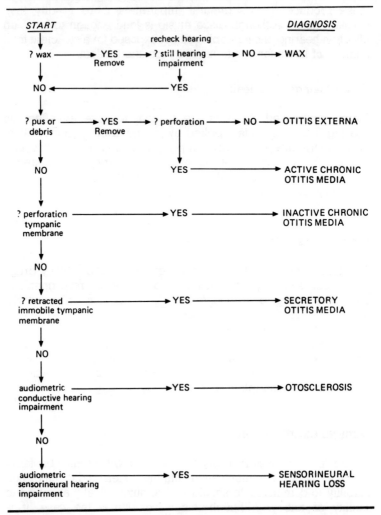

uncertainty as to whether the patient has an impairment or not. This is done by free-field speech testing (page 10). Having confirmed that there is indeed an impairment the next thing to do is examine the ears. *Table 1.2* is a suggested flow pattern used to arrive at a diagnosis.

Are there any operation scars?

This alerts the clinician to the likelihood of the pathology being chronic otitis media and prevents him from automatically ascribing anatomical abnormalities to a disease process.

Is there obstructing wax?

Wax is secreted in the outer third of the canal and though it will frequently obstruct the view of the tympanic membrane it is infrequently the cause of an impairment. This is because sound traverses the external auditory canal as vibrations, not as light does in straight lines, and so provided the wax can vibrate in the column of air it will not cause an impairment. It is only when the wax is impacted into the deeper canal up against the tympanic membrane, most frequently by attempts to clean it out with cotton buds or by the repeated insertion of the mould of a hearing aid that it is likely to cause an impairment (*Figure 1.20*).

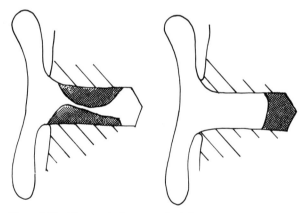

Figure 1.20   The wax in the ear on the left would not cause a hearing impairment whereas the wax on the right would do so

If the tympanic membrane cannot be seen the wax ought to be removed (page 65) because the majority of conductive pathologies are diagnosed by otoscopy. Once the wax has been removed the hearing should be retested, and it is only if the impairment has been eliminated that wax can be said to have been its cause.

Is there any pus, mucus or debris?

If there is any, it has to be removed (page 65) so that a full evaluation can be made. Pus and/or debris in the external auditory canal implies one of two diagnoses. In cases where the skin of the canal is thickened, tender to the examining speculum and produces some degree of canal narrowing, the diagnosis is otitis externa. If there is a tympanic membrane perforation with pus or a mucoid discharge the diagnosis is active chronic otitis media.

A patient may have otitis externa secondary to the pus from active chronic otitis media, so it is vital to visualize the whole area of the tympanic membrane and the attic. To do this requires thorough aural toilet to remove all the pus either by mopping or syringing.

Is the tympanic membrane intact?

Chronic otitis media can, of course, be inactive and there will be no pus or mucus in the canal or middle ear, but there will be a perforation of the tympanic membrane or a defect in the attic. The tympanic membrane may be intact but have white plaques of calcification within it, leading to a diagnosis of tympanosclerosis, which is the end result of any form of otitis media. If the tympanic membrane is intact there remain two relatively common causes of a conductive impairment, otitis media with effusion and otosclerosis. The two are distinguished by the answer to the next question.

Is the tympanic membrane in a normal position and mobile?

In otitis media with effusion the tympanic membrane is usually retracted due to a combination of negative middle ear pressure and the middle ear fluid. To detect this reliably requires considerable experience but is best detected by looking at the handle of the malleus which will be less vertical than normal (*Figure 1.21*). The tympanic membrane itself will look more cone-shaped and perhaps bluish or yellow in colour due to the middle ear fluid.

Another way to diagnose otitis media with effusion is to assess whether the tympanic membrane is mobile. This can be evaluated either dynamically or passively. Watch the tympanic membrane while patient performs a Valsalva manoeuvre (page 8). If the tympanic membrane moves, the Eustachian tube is patent and

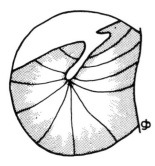

Figure 1.21   Otitis media with effusion. Note the retracted, preshortened handle of the malleus compared with normal (*Figure 1.2*)

there is no fluid in the middle ear. If the tympanic membrane does not move it could be that the patient cannot perform a Valsalva manoeuvre. Positive pressure can then be applied to the external auditory canal by pressing the bulb of a pneumatic otoscope while observing the tympanic membrane. If the tympanic membrane does not move then the diagnosis is otitis media with effusion. Tympanometry (page 16) essentially does the same thing mechanically and can in many cases be helpful in confirming the diagnosis.

What type of hearing impairment is it?

Although the commoner causes of a conductive impairment should have been identified at this stage by otoscopy, tuning fork tests (page 11) can be performed which may help determine whether the impairment has a conductive component to it. However the only way reliably to determine the type and severity of the impairment is by pure tone audiometry. In the presence of a normal external auditory canal and tympanic membrane, a conductive impairment is most likely to be due to otosclerosis, with

Table 1.3 Aetiological factors responsible for sensorineural impairments

Noise trauma
Age (arteriosclerosis)
Ototoxic drugs
Skull fracture
Barotrauma
Viral infections (including mumps and measles)
Labyrinthitis (including Ménière's syndrome)
Acoustic neuroma

congenital abnormalities or ossicular disruption being the alterna-
tives. To distinguish between these is sometimes not easy.

If the impairment is of a sensorineural type, there is little apart
from the history to distinguish between the various aetiological
factors (*Table 3.1*). An important exception is an acoustic neuroma
where further audiometric and radiological tests are of value
(page 50).

How to manage a hearing impairment

Each patient is managed as an individual, and how this is done will
depend on the patient's age, general health, lifestyle, degree of
disability in varying situations, the type of hearing impairment, its
presumed aetiology and the presence of other symptoms. In
general, almost all hearing impairments can be helped by a
hearing aid (page 56) and if there is a conductive component,
surgery may also be of benefit. The next section deals with the
specific management of the few sensorineural conditions that can
be managed and with the surgical management of the commoner
conductive pathologies. The management of any other symptoms
is dealt with elsewhere.

Specific management of hearing in sensorineural impairments

Noise trauma

Impairments due to noise exposure are irreversible, so management is to prevent further exposure. The easiest way to do this is to
avoid excessive noise altogether but this is often impractical
especially for those at work or in the armed forces.

The issue of ear 'defenders' is now compulsory in certain
industries where there is a high level of noise but employees often
pay no heed and go unprotected. There is little evidence that
wearing defenders makes communication with other workers
difficult and this argument for non-wearing should be refuted.
There are many other situations where ear defenders should be
worn. For example, all pneumatic drills and power chain saws
have a high noise output and some tractors and lorry drivers' cabs
are extremely noisy. The crucial factors in the creation of a hearing
loss are the noise level, whether there is sudden impact noise, and
the length of time exposed.

The methods of protection are head muffs or ear plugs (either of insulating cotton, foam or malleable plastic). Ear plugs offer less protection than muffs, and cotton wool is useless.

Ototoxic drugs

As soon as a drug is implicated as being a possible aetiological factor it should be stopped. This applies particularly to the aminoglycosides (gentamicin, kanamycin, streptomycin, etc.) where some recovery of hearing can take place. There should be no difficulty in substituting an alternative drug from a different generic group.

Acoustic neuroma

Surgery, via the ear or the middle or posterior cranial fossa, is necessary to prevent an acoustic neuroma growing and causing intracranial compression. Surgical complications are considerably less for small tumours, so early diagnosis is in the patient's interest. Unfortunately, the hearing usually has to be sacrificed but as the other ear is often normal this is not too disabling.

Specific management of conductive hearing impairments

Chronic otitis media

The tympanic membrane defect can be repaired using fascia or other similar tissue. In appropriate hands, such myringoplasties are highly successful in both improving the hearing and preventing further activity. If the ossicular chain is defective it can be rebuilt using either the patient's own ossicle or a homograft. Artificial prostheses are less satisfactory. Again in the correct hands, such tympanoplasties (i.e. myringoplasty with ossiculo-plasty) can be very beneficial. There is no reason why such operations cannot be carried out in ears that are active but in them the surgical eradication of the inflammation usually takes precedence.

Otosclerosis

In otosclerosis, microsurgery does not remove the pathology but overcomes the stapes fixation by removing it in whole or in part and replacing it with a stainless steel or teflon piston.

In the correct hands, the results are highly satisfactory. The potential complications are a sensorineural impairment, either partial or total, and chronic disequilibrium.

There is no reason why the impairment cannot be managed with a hearing aid.

Otitis media with effusion

Many adults have dullness of hearing for a short period of time following an upper respiratory tract infection. This requires no treatment apart from auto-inflation (Valsalva manoeuvre). In a few patients the condition is chronic, lasting more than three weeks, and the majority of these are idiopathic in origin, perhaps being associated with chronic rhinitis, sinusitus or bronchitis. In a few it is the presenting symptom of a nasopharyngeal tumour, so referral to an otolaryngologist to exclude this is mandatory in those with chronic effusions.

Management is initially medical by any combination of auto-inflation, systemic or topical decongestants and antibiotics. Subsequent surgical management is myringotomy with or without the insertion of a ventilating tube (grommet).

■ Conclusions

- Not all individuals with a hearing impairment are aware that they have one.
- The history is useful in identifying factors which may be responsible for a sensorineural impairment.
- Sensorineural impairments are the commonest type and the commonest aetiological factor is noise exposure.
- Clinical examination should identify the common causes of a conductive impairment, the exception being otosclerosis where the tympanic membrane is normal.

- Although wax often blocks the view of the tympanic membrane, it is an uncommon cause of a hearing impairment.
- The management of a hearing impairment is specific for each patient and depends on its aetiology and the associated disability.
- In general, sensorineural impairments are managed by amplification.
- Conductive hearing impairments can be managed by micro-surgery, amplification, or both.

Hearing impairment in children (otitis media with effusion)

Transient hearing impairments in children are extremely common and in a child who previously had normal hearing, as exemplified by the development of normal speech, there is, in effect, only one likely diagnosis, otitis media with effusion. About one-third of all children will have one or more episodes of otitis media with effusion before they are eight or nine years old, but in the majority these episodes go undetected due to the absence of other symptoms and the relatively minor degree of the impairment. As the majority resolve spontaneously within six weeks and cause no permanent sequelae, the fact that they are missed is of little consequence. However, it is important to identify the 10 per cent or so in whom it does not resolve and in whom the loss is likely to affect their education. This is one of the main reasons that sweep audiometry is carried out in schools in five- to six-year-old children.

Relevant history

Hearing problems in children are very easily missed, so if parents think there is one, they are usually correct. Once a hearing problem has been noticed or brought to the parents' attention they are usually then quite proficient at monitoring variations in the hearing. This is important to know because it is those whose hearing is constantly impaired that cause more concern.

One of the main reasons for managing a child is the potential effect on his education, so the following questions should be asked.

Is the child progressing as well as previously at school? Does the teacher think that the child is not paying attention, when in reality he cannot hear? Is his speech or grammar affected? For example, the child might say 'Daddy dig the garden' missing out the 's' of digs because this is a high frequency consonant which is softly spoken.

It is interesting, and perhaps of some relevance, to find out whether the child has trouble with a blocked nose, mouth breathing and snoring. If present, these might be an indication to progress to adenoidectomy earlier than otherwise.

Clinical examination

The otoscopic diagnosis of otitis media with effusion can be difficult. The commonest finding is retraction of the tympanic membrane, most evident as a retraction of the handle of the malleus which is due to a combination of the middle ear fluid and negative middle ear pressure. The colour of the membrane is often yellowish or bluish, again because of the fluid. Getting a child to perform a Valsalva manoeuvre is probably not worth attempting but in many instances a pneumatic otoscope will help confirm the diagnosis because the tympanic membrane will be immobile.

However, the most important aspect of the clinical examination is to assess the hearing. It takes a certain skill in gaining the cooperation of a child to perform free-field speech tests, and it may require more than one occasion. It is, however, vitally important as the management is based on the results.

Initial non-specialist management

If the child can hear a whispered voice at arm's length in one ear, he is unlikely to suffer any educational consequences. The parents are reassured that resolution is likely but the child is reassessed, say 2–3 months later, to ensure that this is indeed the case.

If the child cannot hear a whispered voice at arm's length in either ear he has to be more carefully managed. It might be hoped that medical therapy would hasten natural resolution but there is little evidence from controlled tests to support the use of systemic decongestants, topical nose drops, mucolytics, antihistamines or antibiotics. The parents often wish the doctor to suggest something, so the child can be encouraged to blow up balloons via his nose rather than his mouth. This is cheap and can be effective but, unfortunately, children soon tire of the game.

School teachers should be informed of the problem to allow them to compensate for the impairment, for example by changing the position of the child in the class.

The waiting period should not be continued for more than 2–3 weeks before the child's hearing is reassessed. If the child again fails the hearing screen, a specialist opinion should be sought.

Specialist management

The first thing that needs to be done by an otolaryngologist is to more accurately assess the hearing by pure tone audiometry. In addition, if the otoscopic findings are uncertain, tympanometry may help in diagnosing otitis media with effusion.

Thereafter, as might be expected, what happens is dependent on who the specialist is. The following might be considered a conservative attitude. Those with bilateral hearing impaired ears are reviewed three months later, and if still impaired, surgery within the next few weeks is suggested.

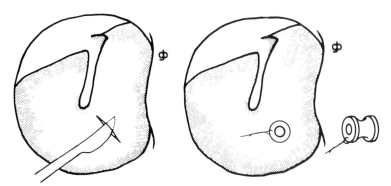

Figure 1.22 Myringotomy (right ear)

Figure 1.23 Grommet inserted in myringotomy slit

Under anaesthesia (usually general anaesthesia in the UK) the middle ear fluid is aspirated through a minute incision (myringotomy) of the tympanic membrane (*Figure 1.22*). Adenoidectomy can be performed at the same time if adenoid hypertrophy is considered to be a contributing factor. The majority of children will have no further hearing problems following myringotomy and aspiration. However, follow-up is essential to identify the few that do have residual hearing problems. In them, repeat myringotomy and aspiration is performed and, in addition, a grommet or ventilation tube is usually inserted (*Figure 1.23*). This equalizes the middle ear pressure with that of the external auditory canal and allows the effusion to drain down the Eustachian tube. The aim is not to drain the fluid into the external auditory canal. The gommmets extrude spontaneously on average six months later and the incision heals. While a grommet is in place the child is often told not to swim, but there is no evidence that swimming increases the incidence of middle ear infection. Some surgeons insert grommets initially but permanent scarring and tympanosclerosis are being increasingly recognized as complications.

■ Conclusions

- In effect, the only diagnosis for a hearing impairment which develops in a previously normal hearing child is otitis media with effusion.
- A considerable number of children with hearing impairments go undetected and routine school screening is designed to detect these.
- The otoscopic diagnosis of otitis media with effusion can be difficult but rests upon the finding of a retracted, immobile tympanic membrane.
- The most important thing is to assess clinically the hearing by free-field voice testing.
- In the majority, otitis media with effusion resolves spontaneously with no sequelae.
- Medical therapy would not appear to hasten this natural resolution.
- Auto-inflation is cheap, does no harm and gives the impression of activity.
- In those that fail to resolve and have a hearing impairment which potentially might impair their education, adenoidectomy along with myringotomy and aspiration is the surgical management.
- A ventilation grommet may be inserted at the same time, but this can cause permanent scarring of the tympanic membrane.

Hearing impairment in infants

Unfortunately, hearing impairments in infants often go unrecognized, and because of the resultant sensory deprivation they can develop speech, educational and psychological problems. The main aim of those involved must be to identify infants with an impairment as early as possible so that their residual hearing can be aided by amplification and hopefully with this the child will develop normal speech and be able to lead a relatively normal life.

An infant may be either born with a hearing impairment or may acquire it early in life. When the impairment is present at birth it can be prenatal, perinatal or postnatal in origin. Such impairments will not be obvious at birth, so it is necessary to look for them. Overall the risk is about 1 per 1000 births so for practical reasons more, but not exclusive, attention is paid to infants particularly at risk, for example, because of prematurity, prolonged labour or jaundice.

Prenatal

The vast majority of infants with a genetically determined hearing impairment have no obvious congenital defect and are thus not so easy to detect as the smaller group in which the impairment is part of a syndrome complex with multiple, often visible, defects (e.g. Treacher–Collins and Down's syndrome). Children of deaf parents are obviously more at risk but in the majority, the impairment can only be attributed to spontaneous mutations.

It is normally assumed that a hearing impairment present at birth is genetic if there are no obvious other factors.

The most important non-genetic, prenatal aetiology is rubella virus infection (german measles) of the mother during the first 12 weeks of pregnancy. This is the time during which the fetal ear (otocyst) is developing and is, therefore, particularly at risk. At present, rubella cannot be treated, but it is currently recommended that all 14-year-old girls should be immunized unless they already have high antibody titres.

Viruses other than rubella have also been suggested as a cause but the evidence for this is not convincing. Drugs taken during pregnancy can cause fetal abnormalities including a hearing impairment and should, therefore, be avoided whenever possible.

Perinatal factors

Hypoxia during birth mainly affects neurological structures and the premature underweight infant is particularly at risk. Hence spastics, the end result of perinatal hypoxia, are prone both to being mentally defective and having a hearing impairment.

Jaundice in the fetus is particularly damaging, both to the brain and the hearing, due to the neurotoxicity of the bilirubin. Infants with jaundice at birth, either from haemolytic disease (Rh incompatibility) or due to prematurity should, therefore, be observed with particular care.

Postnatal factors

Postnatal sensorineural impairments are most often caused by one of three infections: mumps, measles or meningitis. Of these meningitis is associated with a higher incidence of bilateral, severe impairments so all children should have their hearing tested once they have recovered from the meningitis. Some consider that subclinical infection by mumps or measles viruses may also be responsible for a number of cases when no other factor can be identified.

How do you identify an infant with a hearing impairment?

Newborn babies are difficult to assess but future developments of computerized 'cradles' that record the child's movements in reaction to repeated sound stimuli may solve this problem. Brain stem evoked response audiometry is a more sophisticated alternative (page 16).

In Britain it is routine for all children to be visited at home by a health visitor for developmental checks which include the hearing. In most instances the mother will recognize that there is something wrong in the first months of life, when the child does not respond to her voice. In addition, at this age children should be beginning to say monosyllables such as 'ba' and 'da'. Startle reflex testing of infants is too uncertain to be relied upon. It is only when children are six to seven months old that they can be screened by using distraction tests. These are random noises, preferably generated from a portable sound box, which are presented out of sight while the child's attention is being held. The hearing child should turn in response to the sounds. As can be imagined, this is liable to misinterpretation and whenever there is any doubt evoked response audiometry should be performed.

Children who are not saying bisyllables such as 'papa' and 'mama', etc. by the age of nine months should be considered to have a hearing impairment. Even mentally defective children should achieve this and articulation defects without any other evidence of spasticity should not preclude this achievement.

By the age of 18–30 months a normally hearing child should be able to perform cooperation tests such as responding to 'where are your shoes?'. Only when the child is about 30 months old is it possible to do performance tests such as play audiometry, in which the child is taught to perform a task such as putting a brick on a pile when he hears a sound. As can be imagined, there are many children, especially those with multiple defects, in whom there is no clear answer. For them, objective tests of hearing, including evoked response audiometry, are increasingly being used.

Having identified an impairment, what do you do?

Even though the impairment may have a conductive component due to a congenital abnormality of the external or middle ear, the initial management in all cases is amplification with a hearing aid and specialized education as soon as the impairment is detected. Special high power aids are usually necessary. Acceptance of the wearing of these is better in infants than in school-age children.

As the main aim is to integrate deaf children into the community, the trend is to have a special class for the deaf in a normal school if it is not possible to integrate the child totally into a normal class, rather than to have separate schools for the deaf.

■ Conclusions

- It is vital to diagnose hearing impairments in infants early so that the resultant speech, communication, educational and psychological handicap can be mitigated by amplification and intensive education.

- It is better to over-suspect and thereby not miss an infant with an impairment rather than to underdiagnose.
- Audiometric testing is difficult in infants, and increasing reliance is being placed on objective methods such as evoked response audiometry.

Unilateral sensorineural hearing impairment

The presence of a hearing impairment in only one ear, or the presence of a hearing impairment more severe in one ear than the other, is relatively common in individuals with a conductive hearing impairment. Such impairments usually present no diagnostic problem.

What is less common is a unilateral or an asymmetric sensorineural hearing impairment. It is important to identify these because one of the causes, albeit a rare one, is an acoustic neuroma of the VIII cranial nerve in the internal auditory canal. Although these are benign fibromas of the nerve sheath, if left untreated they can expand outside the canal and cause death by pressing on the brain stem. It is, therefore, important to identify an acoustic neuroma as early as possible so that it can be surgically removed.

The main differential diagnoses of known causes of a unilateral or asymmetric sensorineural hearing impairment apart from an acoustic neuroma are measles, mumps, meningitis, trauma (head injury, barotrauma or surgery), asymmetric noise exposure and ototoxic antibiotics. These can all usually be fairly easily diagnosed from the history.

There remains a large idiopathic group in which the cause is unknown. It is important that before a patient is included in this idiopathic group an acoustic neuroma is excluded. This can only be done by specialized audiometric tests or radiology. As such, all individuals with a unilateral sensorineural hearing impairment without an obvious cause should be referred to an otolaryngologist for screening. The incidence of acoustic neuroma in such individuals will be low, but the benefit of early diagnosis is great in terms of reduced postoperative morbidity.

■ Conclusions

- Conductive hearing impairments are often unilateral or asymmetric.
- Sensorineural unilateral or asymmetric hearing impairments are relatively uncommon but all those without an obvious cause from the history should be referred to exclude an acoustic neuroma.

Sudden hearing loss

Sudden deteriorations in hearing should be considered an otological emergency, as the diagnosis is best made by a specialist during the acute episode. Only the specialist can distinguish accurately between a conductive and a sensorineural impairment. Specialist monitoring is also important because, in the case of barotrauma, surgical management may be deemed necessary. In general, a considerable proportion (70 per cent) will recover spontaneously but it is the remaining 30 per cent who should concern us. At present there is no way of identifying who will and who will not recover, so it is necessary to see all individuals with sudden hearing loss as soon as possible.

Most suddent hearing losses are unilateral but occasionally they are bilateral. Vertigo is usually also present but may only be mild.

Known causes

The aetiological factors responsible for sudden hearing loss have not all been identified. Those that are recognized can usually be identified from the history (*Table 1.4*) supplemented occasionally by clinical findings. Once all the known factors have been excluded the aetiology is a matter for conjecture.

Water/wax

Water loading the tympanic membrane and unable to get out because of wax should be easy to diagnose and correct if it does not resolve spontaneously. The impaction of wax with a cotton bud can also cause a sudden loss.

Table 1.4 Diagnosis of sudden hearing loss

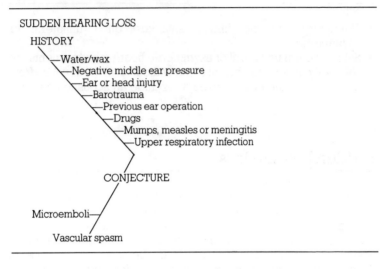

SUDDEN HEARING LOSS
HISTORY
—Water/wax
—Negative middle ear pressure
—Ear or head injury
—Barotrauma
—Previous ear operation
—Drugs
—Mumps, measles or meningitis
—Upper respiratory infection

CONJECTURE

Microemboli—
Vascular spasm

Negative middle ear pressure/early otitis media with effusion

Many individuals will develop negative middle ear pressure because of Eustachian tube dysfunction associated with a cold. If persistent, early otitis media with effusion will develop. The diagnosis is made by the association with a cold, a history of previous episodes, the inability to auto-inflate the ear(s) and otoscopy. The hearing impairment is minimal and self-resolving.

Barotrauma

When the Eustachian tube is not functioning properly in association with an upper respiratory tract infection, the problems are never severe. It is a different matter, however, when there are extreme changes of pressure such as in a poorly pressurized aeroplane or when diving. The pressure in the middle ear is then grossly different from that in the inner ear. The Eustachian tube does not allow pressure equalization and the round window membrane may rupture, causing a perilymph fistula which results in a sudden sensorineural hearing loss. A history of recent air travel or diving should, therefore, always be enquired about when there is a sudden hearing loss. There is almost invariably associated vertigo, which may not be complained of because it can be mild.

The treatment of a sudden sensorineural hearing loss due to barotrauma is admission to hospital for bedrest and daily audiometric monitoring of the hearing. If the loss is severe or progressing, surgical closure of the fistula may be indicated.

Previous ear operation

In a patient with a sudden hearing loss it is important to ascertain whether there has been a previous operation on the affected ear.

Ears in which the oval window has been opened, as in a stapedectomy, are particularly at risk of developing a perilymph fistula in the same manner as in barotrauma, but at the oval rather than the round window. In these circumstances there need be no great pressure change; a cough is all that is required to cause a break. The management is surgical sealing of the oval window.

Ear and head injuries

Such injuries can cause either a sensorineural loss due to inner ear damage or a conductive hearing loss due to middle ear bleeding with or without ossicular chain disruption (page 170). A conductive impairment may particularly benefit from surgery.

Drugs

The aminoglycosides (streptomycin, kanamycin, tobramycin, gentamicin) and diuretics (especially those administered intravenously) are particularly ototoxic and as many of these drugs are excreted by the kidneys, patients with renal failure are especially at risk. Once a sufficient concentration of the drug is achieved in the perilymph the hair cells are damaged, thus producing a sensorineural hearing loss which is most commonly bilateral but can be unilateral. Monitoring of serum levels can help to reduce the incidence of ototoxicity but should a patient develop a hearing loss, tinnitus or vertigo while on any drug, it should be stopped immediately unless necessary for life. Thereafter, the hearing should be monitored, as the hearing loss can still progress because of selective concentration of the drug in the inner ear.

Mumps, measles, meningitis

These three relatively common infections of childhood are recognized to cause neuritis, and the commonest single cranial nerve to be affected is the VIII nerve. Fortunately this complication is relatively rare and often on one side only. The sensorineural hearing loss often goes unrecognized at the time and there is no proven management, although steroids have been suggested. It is unlikely that subclinical mumps or measles is a common cause of sudden hearing loss but if either is suspected serial antibody titres at the time will aid the diagnosis.

Upper respiratory tract and renal infections

Sudden sensorineural hearing losses are often attributed to a recent cold or influenza. On occasions this may be the case but, considering the high incidence of upper respiratory tract infections in the population at any one time, it is not surprising that individuals with a sudden hearing loss often have such a history.

Idiopathic sensorineural causes

Having excluded the known causes from the history, the clinician is often left to conjecture the aetiology of the sudden hearing loss. The most commonly postulated factors are all vascular and it would seem highly probable that, as the inner ear is supplied by an end artery, thrombosis, microemboli or spasm can be responsible. However, unless there is evidence of such pathology in other organs, there is no way of confirming this suspicion. Vascular dilators, anticoagulants and steroids have all been suggested and tried in patients with an idiopathic loss with variable results.

■ Conclusions

- Individuals with a sudden hearing loss should be referred for a specialist opinion as soon as possible.
- The known aetiological factors are best identified from the history.

- Sudden hearing loss caused by changes in atmospheric pressure and previous surgery often benefit from early surgery.

Fluctuating hearing

Outer and middle ear causes of fluctuating hearing are more common than inner ear causes. If there is not an obvious cause in the outer ear, the differentiation can be difficult and require a specialist opinion and audiometry.

Outer ear causes

Wax and otitis externa can cause a varying hearing impairment due to varying degrees of occlusion of the external auditory canal. The diagnosis should be obvious on otoscopy.

A temporary impairment due to water immobilizing the tympanic membrane after showering, or bathing, is common.

Middle ear causes

Many people experience a feeling of fullness or dullness in their ears during or following an upper respiratory tract infection. This is caused by Eustachian tube malfunction creating a negative middle ear pressure which may be followed by a small middle ear effusion. The ears look relatively normal and the hearing impairment is so minor that it usually cannot be audiometrically detected. If the impairment is helped by auto-inflation, the diagnosis is confirmed and treatment effected.

The hearing impairment associated with chronic otitis media can also vary and is often least when the ear is actively discharging because the mucopus bridges any defects in the ossicular chain or tympanic membrane. The diagnosis should be evident on otoscopy and the management is as described elsewhere (page 26).

Inner ear causes

These are extremely rare and the mechanism is often difficult to define. If the episodes of decreased hearing are associated with vertigo and there is no obvious cause, it is called Ménière's syndrome. At present there is no proven medical or surgical treatment specific to Ménière's syndrome (page 73).

■ Conclusions

- Fluctuating hearing due to wax, otitis externa and chronic otitis media are common, but perhaps the commest cause is Eustachian tube malfunction following an upper respiratory tract infection.
- Fluctuating sensorineural hearing impairments are rare. Ménière's syndrome is the symptom complex of episodic vertigo with fluctuating (sensorineural) hearing.

Hearing aids for the hearing impaired

One must be highly critical of advertisers who imply that all one need do is to walk into their premises and buy a hearing aid. Hearing aids can be of considerable benefit but there are three main reasons why a commercial purchase should not be done initially: medical, financial and rehabilitation.

An otologist should always be consulted because a conductive hearing impairment can often be helped by surgery, though this is not the management in every case. Though sensorineural impairments cannot at present be helped by surgery, such impairments can be the portent of more serious disease, such as an acoustic neuroma. A doctor is the only person trained to recognize such conditions and his timely recognition and treatment could prevent serious complications.

In Britain and several European and Commonwealth countries, hearing aids are provided through the Health Services, either free or at a considerably reduced cost. In the first instance, then, it would be financially sound to try a Health Service aid to assess its benefit. If it is of minimal or no benefit, then it is unlikely that a commercial aid would be any better. If it is of benefit, then a commercial aid might be worth considering as there are a larger variety of designs available with different aesthetic qualities, such as 'in-the-ear' and 'in-the-canal' aids. If the purchase of a commercial aid is subsequently considered, the Health Service aid will form a basis for comparison and it is unlikely that a poor buy will be made.

Finally, but not least, are the follow-up services that only an otologist's team can provide. Many people experience great difficulty in using their aids and follow-up and rehabilitation are perhaps best done when the service is free or at least when included in the cost of a private hearing aid.

Who might benefit from a hearing aid?

The answer to this question is anyone with a hearing impairment that makes him sufficiently disabled to be motivated to learn to use one.

The types of situation in which a patient has difficulty in hearing equates fairly closely with his degree of impairment so that a mild impairment will make it difficult to hear in a noisy background. With moderate impairments the volume of the television has to be raised and understanding speech in quiet conditions will be a problem, but how much a patient is disabled will depend considerably on his ability to speech read. With severe and profound impairments, background noises will not be heard at all and understanding speech will depend entirely on speech reading.

Unfortunately, the wearing of a hearing aid is not as simple as wearing a pair of glasses. Hearing aids do not return the hearing to normal, mainly because they are amplification systems of low fidelity which boost all sounds to the same extent whether these sounds are speech or background noise. In those with a sensorineural impairment there is, in addition to a loss of volume, a loss of frequency discrimination which makes speech difficult to comprehend. For this reason, individuals with a conductive impairment benefit more from an aid than those with a comparable sensorineural impairment. Individual patients will also differ in how much benefit they get from an aid and all will find some circumstances where it is more of a hindrance than a help. Many will also find the physical aspects of using an aid daunting, in particular, inserting the mould, so unless the patient and his professional advisors are motivated to pursue the wearing of an aid then it will not be worn.

What types of aids are available?

Behind-the-ear aids

These suffer from the disadvantages of:

1. Wind noise.
2. Feedback noise if the patient does not insert the mould correctly or if it fits poorly.
3. Sometimes older fingers find the volume control difficult to adjust in comparison to a body-worn aid.

They have the advantage of:

1. Appearance.

'In-the-ear' and 'in-the-canal' aids

These suffer from the disadvantages of:

1. Cost. They are much dearer than behind-the-ear aids and are not available through the UK National Health Service.
2. Lack of volume. This is mainly due to feedback which limits the gain that can be used.
3. Lack of fidelity.

They have the advantage of:

1. Appearance. This is mainly a psychological one created by good commercial marketing. It could be argued that a behind-the-ear aid is less noticeable particularly if the wearer has hair.

Body-worn aids

These suffer from the disadvantages of:

1. Appearance.
2. Noise from clothes rub.

They have the advantages of:

1. Easy adjustment because of relatively easy access and visibility.
2. Considerable amplification potential which can be used because of the absence of feedback.

Bone-conduction aids

Bone-conduction aids are mainly used where an actively discharging ear precludes the use of an ear mould. Their use has now been almost obviated by the good results of surgery for chronic otitis media and of topical medications for otitis externa.

What types of ear moulds are available?

Personal moulds

1. Standard (Figure 1.24). The ear canal is completely occluded by these moulds, lessening feedback of amplified sound to the aid's microphone, which can be a problem especially with high powered ear-level aids. Feedback is evident by screeching of the aid when it is in the ear.

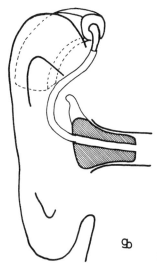

Figure 1.24   Ear-level aid with standard mould

2. Ventilated. These have the potential advantage of overcoming the blocked-up feeling of a closed mould and of amplifying more selectively the high frequencies which may benefit those with a high tone sensorineural impairment. Their disadvantage is that they are more prone to feedback, so they can only be used with mild impairments where there is less need to turn up

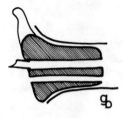

Figure 1.25   Ventilated ear mould

the volume. A ventilation hole can be drilled in a standard mould (*Figure 1.25*) or, alternatively there may be no mould in the canal, the tube being held at the entrance to the canal by a special earpiece.

Temporary moulds

These are available in a variety of sizes and may be issued during a trial period. They consist either of a flanged plastic bung or of an acrylic mould and their use is discontinued once a personal mould has been made.

How is an aid prescribed?

Once it has been decided to prescribe an aid several factors have to be considered. For cosmetic reasons, patients want ear-level rather than body-worn aids. This should be complied with, but patients with poor finger dexterity may require a body-worn aid.

Patients with a mild to moderate, bilateral hearing impairment are often reluctant to be fitted with two aids and it is usual to fit a monaural aid to the poorer hearing ear, if there is one. If the hearing is equal in both ears then the choice can be left to the patient who often finds the non-telephone ear preferable as he does not have to take the aid out to use the telephone.

Patients with a bilateral, severe impairment should be persuaded to try two aids but if they only wish for one it should be fitted to the better hearing ear.

The switch with the three positions 'O', 'T' and 'M' is explained: '**O**' for 'Off'; '**T**' for use with a **T**elecoil accessory aid (see below); '**M**' for '**M**icrophone on'. The ability to control the volume of the output by the wheel is explained and it is emphasized that the level of amplification will have to be varied in different circumstances and not kept at a particular setting.

An impression is made of the patient's ear and this is used to make the personal mould. At this time the opportunity is taken to give advice which might help the patient cope better with his hearing impairment. Thus speech reading classes might be suggested and the availability of attachments which amplify the television, radio and telephone mentioned.

Is there a need for follow-up?

Once a hearing aid has been prescribed, it is essential to see the patient again to ascertain whether he or she is having any difficulties. The majority will initially have problems particularly in inserting the ear mould. The problems can usually all be solved, although often a great deal of patience and understanding has to be displayed with the elderly.

Inability to insert the ear mould

It is astonishing how many patients cannot insert the ear mould because they don't know which way it goes in. Even more have difficulty in inserting the anti-tragal part, which can lead to non-use because of feedback and skin ulceration (*Figure 1.26*). So at the

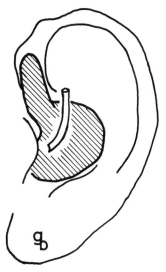

Figure 1.26   Incorrectly inserted ear mould

return visit every recipient should demonstrate that he or she can insert the mould correctly, switch the aid on and control the volume.

Feedback

Feedback is the screeching sound produced by the microphone picking up and amplifying the sound that it is putting out. The commonest cause for feedback is a poorly fitting mould, either because the mould itself is poorly made or because the patient has not put it in correctly. Moulds deteriorate with time and the patient's ear and canal can change with ageing so renewal of ear moulds is frequently necessary. This is especially necessary with a high powered aid as feedback can be more of a problem with this type.

Too noisy

Naturally, if one has not heard traffic and other background noise for some time the cerebral processes which normally exclude these from consciousness have to be relearned. In addition, many individuals have to be reminded that the volume has to be frequently adjusted in different circumstances.

Can't be bothered

Adaptation to an aid requires time and perseverance. Many of the elderly do not exhibit the latter and in them it is usually the relatives that want to be heard rather than the patient who wants to hear. Counselling the relatives is probably the most sensible solution.

Aid broken or not working

First ensure that the mould is not blocked with wax; it needs frequent cleaning with soap and water and occasionally with a nailbrush. Next make sure the parts of the aid are properly connected and that the tube is not twisted. Switch the aid on. If there is no feedback at full volume, the battery is likely to be flat. With a body-worn aid excess noise and crackling suggest that the wires in the lead are broken or loose.

■ Conclusions

- As there may be something more seriously wrong and as surgery might be able to help, individuals with a hearing impairment should always see an otologist before being provided with an aid.
- Hearing aids can be of considerable benefit so if in doubt in an individual nothing is lost by trying one out.
- How much benefit a patient will gain from an aid is a combination of his or her disability, speech reading skills and motivation.
- Hearing aids are often not used because of insufficient explanation regarding the insertion of the ear mould and the use of the aid.
- All patients who are provided with an aid should be followed-up to ensure that they can perform all the practical tasks associated with using an aid.
- Feedback can be a reason for lack of benefit but this can be overcome by ensuring that the mould fits well and is correctly inserted.
- Hearing aids and the mould need to be maintained.
- Look out for the situation where it is the relatives rather than the patient who want an aid.
- There are few reasons why a commercial aid should be purchased in preference to an NHS aid.

Accessory aids for the hearing impaired

The natural inclination is to fit a hearing aid and forget that for many individuals accessory aids can be of equal if not more value.

The disability that an individual experiences with a given impairment is dependent on his lifestyle. For example, someone living alone might have the greatest difficulty listening to the television. If there are no complaining neighbours he just turns up the volume, but if there are it might be better to suggest a television head-set rather than a hearing aid.

There are a wide variety of accessory aids available on the commercial market but they can be categorized into three types according to usage:

With a television
With a telephone
Bells

In Britain at present, these aids are not available from the National Health Service, but in certain circumstances financial aid can be given through the local Social Services Department.

Some of these aids use an induction loop. This is a circuit of wire into which the sound is passed electrically. This will set up, by induction, a similar electrical signal within a coil which is in the hearing aid. This is switched on by setting the hearing aid to the 'T' (telecoil) position. A loop system has the advantages of allowing the user to move around unattached to a wire and of excluding background sounds which may otherwise be troublesome. Their main disadvantage is that they pick up other electrical sounds. Loop systems can be fitted in public halls, theatres and churches as well as being used with television and the telephone.

Television aids

These can be particularly useful, especially when there are other individuals in the room who do not appreciate a loud television set. Most sets have a socket for these aids but if not they can usually be attached by a television engineer.

There are two alternative types of aid. The first is where there is a direct output to headphones or to an ear mould. The second type uses an induction loop system; the most popular model has a loop of wire from the television in a cushion which is placed on the seat where the user sits to watch the television.

Telephone aids

The two main methods of amplification are by increasing the volume on the handset or by using a loop system. The handset can have a volume control built into it but this restricts the user to such phones. Alternatively, an amplifier can be carried around and fitted over any handset. To use the telecoil in a patient's aid requires the phone to be fitted with an induction coil.

Telephone and door bells

Hard of hearing individuals are often concerned that they cannot hear the telephone or door bell. There are several solutions. The first is to change the position of the bell to a more suitable location, such as from the hall to the sitting room. The second is to get a louder bell and preferably one with a low frequency output, as most individuals with a hearing impairment are particularly affected at the higher frequencies. Flashing lights are only necessary for the profoundly hard of hearing. The final, very effective alternative, is to buy a 'wee dug' (small dog).

■ Conclusions

- Accessory aids can often be of as much value to a patient as a hearing aid.
- It is important in any individual case to take into acount what difficulties he or she is having before coming to a decision as to the type of aid.

Ear syringing

When examining an ear, the view of the tympanic membrane will often be obstructed by wax. If the patient has otological symptoms the wax has to be removed as conductive pathologies are mainly diagnosed by otoscopy. If the patient has no symptoms the wax does not need to be removed. On the other hand pus and/or debris has always to be removed both to manage the condition and to diagnose the responsible pathology. Pus can be mopped away but it is often quicker to syringe it out. The method of syringing is the same, irrespective of what is being removed, but, for clarity, the removal of wax will be described.

If the wax is soft, it can be syringed out immediately but if impacted it can be loosened by inserting a probe under direct vision between the canal wall and the wax. Once disimpaction or partial removal has been achieved, any remains are syringed out. The alternative is wax softening which can take several days, and may make the obstructive symptoms temporarily worse. This method, however, is easier if the clinician is inexperienced at using a probe. Expensive proprietary wax softeners are not necessary, and can act as skin irritants. Sodium bicarbonate ear drops BPC are as effective and cheaper, and there is nothing wrong with olive or almond oil.

In syringing, the object is to syringe water past the wax up to the drum, where it will be outwardly displaced, bringing the wax with it. Waterproof drapes are essential for the patient and for inexperienced operators. Whether the syringe is made of metal, plastic or rubber is irrelevant provided it has a blunt tip to avoid traumatizing the canal. The syringe is filled with tap water at body temperature – higher or lower temperatures can cause vertigo due to an unwanted caloric response. The canal is first straightened by pulling the pinna posterosuperiorly, and the water is directed against the posterosuperior canal wall, where there is usually a gap between it and the wax. Progress should be checked regularly by direct inspection and after completion the canal must be dried with cotton buds. Thereafter, the ear must be inspected. Gross damage is uncommon but there is usually temporary hyperaemia of the drum and canal due to the syringing.

As stated earlier syringing is one of the best methods for clearing pus and debris from the external canal as well as from mastoid cavities. The presence of infection is not a contraindication, as the middle ear is already infected. The only relative contraindication to syringing is an ear with known inactive chronic otitis media and a perforation. Even here, the chance of introducing infection is minimal if an aseptic technique is adopted and meticulous mopping performed thereafter.

■ Conclusions

- Large amounts of soft wax or pus and debris are probably most easily removed by syringing, especially by the inexperienced operator.

- Small amounts of wax are probably removed quicker with a cotton bud under direct vision.
- Impacted hard wax can be softened with olive oil, almond oil or sodium bicarbonate ear drops BPC before syringing. Alternatively, wax may be loosened under direct vision with a probe.
- The presence of infection is not a contraindication to syringing.
- Similarly, perforation of the tympanic membrane is not a contraindication to syringing.
- The ear should always be dried and examined after syringing.

Noises in the ear (tinnitus)

Tinnitus can be a very alarming symptom, some patients considering it to be the first sign of mental illness. Certainly, if the noises speak to them, they are probably correct, but otherwise patients can be reassured that it is a relatively common symptom and not a portent of mental illness, strokes or intracranial tumours.

There are two types of tinnitus. The first is otological (subjective) tinnitus, which only the patient can hear, and is usually ascribed to cochlear malfunction. This type of tinnitus is common, affecting at some time or other about 15 per cent of the population. Thankfully, the vast majority of patients are not troubled by it. The second type is transmitted tinnitus, which sometimes the doctor can hear, and is usually caused by an abnormal arterial blood flow. This type is comparatively rare and, as it usually has a beating quality, can be identified by asking the question 'Does the noise beat?'.

Otological or subjective tinnitus

Otological tinnitus is often likened to a high pitched hiss or running water and is not usually pulsatile. The severity of the tinnitus can vary from day to day, but it is most often noticed in quiet surroundings and hence can be particularly troublesome in the evening when it is quiet or when the patient is trying to sleep.

This tinnitus is normally associated with a hearing loss, although this can be so slight as not to have been noticed by the patient.

Pathophysiologically, tinnitus is considered to be an inappropriate discharge from damaged hair cells or acoustic nerve fibres, but as tinnitus is just as common in conductive as in sensorineural hearing impairments, this is not the only answer.

In a patient, the main thing to assess is the degree of distress that the tinnitus is causing. The majority of individuals adjust well to their tinnitus and need no management apart from reassurance. On the other hand, there are some patients who will be depressed, but in them it is the depression that is the primary illness which requires management rather than the other way round.

Naturally, if a specific otological disease is identified which requires a hearing aid or surgery, this is recommended, and the resultant improvement in hearing, by introducing previously unheard background sounds, may reduce the awareness of the tinnitus. If the otological disease does not require treatment the tinnitus can be managed in a variety of ways but unfortunately, at present there are no specific anti-tinnitus drugs which are of proven value.

Management

1. Reassure the patient that tinnitus is not a portent of mental illness or brain disease, and that it usually becomes less troublesome with time. The majority of individuals will need nothing further.
2. Masking the tinnitus with another noise can be particularly useful in the evening or at night when the patient will be more aware of his tinnitus because there is little else to occupy his mind. Background music/speech or interstation noise from a radio or TV can be useful. In bed, to avoid disturbing a sleeping partner, a transistor radio can be put under the pillow.
3. Tinnitus maskers look like an ear-level aid but produce a background noise which many patients find to be of considerable psychological support.
4. Tranquillizers or antidepressants may be prescribed but only where considered relevant.
5. Night sedation can be prescribed.

Transmitted tinnitus

In the patient who has pulsatile tinnitus, the source can sometimes be elicited by listening over the neck for carotid artery bruits or transmitted murmurs from the heart. The skull can be listened over for an arteriovenous fistula and the ear can be looked into for a glomus jugulare tumour. This can often be seen as a bluish pulsation behind the tympanic membrane and can be associated with cranial nerve palsies (particularly IX, X, XI and XII) due to compression by the tumour as they pass through the skull foramina.

■ Conclusions

- Tinnitus is a common symptom, mainly otological in origin.
- It is usually associated with a hearing impairment, either conductive or sensorineural.
- The hearing impairment should be managed on its own account as improving the hearing can introduce previously unheard background noise which masks the tinnitus.
- The majority of patients will learn to accept the tinnitus if reassured that it is not a portent of serious disease.
- Many find the use of background noise/music in the evening or when trying to get to sleep a useful distraction.
- A tinnitus masker is an alternative source of distracting noise.
- Some patients who are depressed complain vociferously about their tinnitus. In them antidepressant medication is indicated.
- Transmitted tinnitus from a vascular abnormality is relatively uncommon and the source may be detected by auscultation.

Disequilibrium

Most clinicians feel uncomfortable when faced with a patient with balance problems. This is partly because investigations are usually of minimal benefit in arriving at a diagnosis, making the clinician rely heavily on clinical judgement. Indeed, in the majority of individuals, no definite diagnosis will be made. Fortunately, this is not too important as the management is the same for most – reassurance that the disability will lessen with time and, if considered necessary, the prescription of one of various sedatives.

Applied neurophysiology

The clinician's first task is to elucidate the symptoms and decide the most appropriate syndrome complex the patient has. This will help to decide whether their origin is primarily otological, central or both. To understand this distinction a working knowledge of the neurophysiology is necessary.

The brain stem, acting as the coordinating centre, receives a sensory input from the eyes, from the limbs and from the vestibular system of the two ears (*Figure 1.27*). The cerebellum coordinates

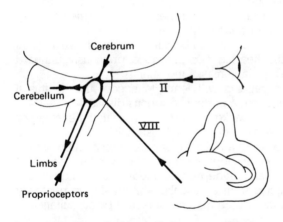

Figure 1.27   Neurophysiology of balance control

body movements in response to these sensory inputs and the cerebrum exerts some overall control. Take any one of the sensory inputs away, for example by shutting the eyes, and the system will still function well. Provide a faulty or contradictory input from one and disequilibrium occurs. A common physiological cause of disequilibrium is sea sickness, when the horizon is not visually horizontal. The visual position of the waves does not tally with the input from the semicircular canals or the limbs and disequilibrium will then occur if the cerebellum cannot compensate.

Disease in any part or parts of the system can cause

disequilibrium. Eye disease is not discussed further because of its rarity, and proprioceptor disease is not discussed as it should be readily identified by the associated problems of controlling the limbs.

What are the patient's symptoms and what syndrome is he most likely to have?

In the majority of individuals with disequilibrium it is the history that enables a diagnosis to be made but this takes time and is not easy. It is far better to take time with finding the history rather than investigating the patient as the investigation is seldom of great value. What actually happens during an episode of disequilibrium is the first thing to enquire about and in general the patient will complain of one of the following.

Vertigo. This is the sensation of rotation, either of the patient or his surroundings and is often accompanied by nausea and occasionally vomiting. Those who have drunk alcohol to excess will probably recognize the symptoms, especially the fact that the symptoms are made worse by shutting the eyes. Vertigo is most frequently a result of otological pathology, but not all otological pathology causes vertigo. The first episode of vertigo tends to be the worst and if there are any subsequent episodes these tend to be less severe because the system compensates.

Lightheadedness. This symptom has no need of a description but it is important to know whether lightheadedness occurs on changing the body's position as the patient can be advised to do this more slowly. The most likely cause is postural hypotension which occurs when the body's pressure receptors are unable to respond fast enough to a change in posture, most notably on getting up from a sitting or lying posture. Typically, the patient has lightheadedness only when getting up and the effect is mitigated by getting up more slowly. Hypotensive medication for hypertension does not help postural hypotension. Any drug, in fact, can cause lightheadedness, including those prescribed for disequilibrium. This is one of the easier diagnoses to prove as the cessation of medication or changing to a different pharmacological group of drugs should relieve the symptoms.

Imbalance. This typically only occurs on movement, the patient often staggering to one side in particular. There are many causes for this, not least the general incoordination which goes with ageing. Most patients with imbalance usually have non-otological problems but otological disease, in the acute stage, can cause imbalance. This tends to be compensated for with time whereas central causes do not.

Blackouts/falls. The patient will usually have no difficulty in deciding whether he temporarily loses consciousness, falls to the ground, or both. Such a history will rule out otological conditions as being responsible.

Having elucidated what form the disequilibrium takes, the clinician has then to decide by further questioning which symptom complex the patient is most likely to have. At this stage it is worth stating what these complexes are, particularly as clinical examination and laboratory investigation will be helpful in only a few cases.

Otological syndromes and conditions causing disequilibrium

Acute labyrinthine dysfunction

This has a typical presentation. The vertigo is prostrating and can take several days to settle. There may or may not be auditory symptoms but there is invariably spontaneous nystagmus. The cause in most cases is unknown. The identifiable causes are all traumatic; head injury, barotrauma or surgery. The remainder are suggested to be due to viral infections either of the vestibular nerve or of the labyrinth. In most, the system gradually compensates and there is no further trouble. If the problem continues, subsequent episodes become progressively less severe and less frequent, and will usually disappear completely after 12–18 months.

Chronic labyrinthine dysfunction

The episodes last minutes rather than days and are not grossly disabling because the system has learned to compensate. There may or may not be an associated hearing impairment or tinnitus. There are four recognized subgroups which will account for most, but not all, patients with chronic labyrinthine dysfunction.

Chronic otitis media   can cause vestibular dysfunction either by extension of the infection into the vestibular labyrinth or by erosion of the bone covering the lateral semicircular canal.

Positional vertigo   is characterized by sudden, relatively short episodes of vertigo which only occur when the head is in certain positions. It occurs whether the neck is hyperextended or not and is thus differentiated from vertebrobasilar ischaemia (*see below*). Positional vertigo can be confirmed by positional testing (*see* page 75).

Acoustic neuromas   are neurofibromas of the vestibular nerve which, although simple tumours, can cause death by pressing on the brain stem. It is, therefore, important to diagnose them early to enable surgical removal with as little neurological damage as possible. Acoustic neuromas have a variable presentation but almost invariably there is a unilateral hearing impairment. Disequilibrium is not common because the growth of the tumour is so slow that compensation occurs. It is important, however, to screen all patients with disequilibrium to identify whether they have a unilateral hearing impairment.

Ménière's syndrome   is the symptom complex of episodic vertigo and fluctuating sensorineural hearing impairment which may or may not be accompanied by tinnitus and fullness in the ear(s). Like most vestibular problems the vertigo usually becomes progressively less severe and frequent but the hearing impairment may become permanent. Ménière's syndrome is relatively rare, although the title is often erroneously ascribed to any dizzy patient. There is no proven specific management, either medical or surgical, for this syndrome.

Non-otological conditions causing disequilibrium

Ageing

This is perhaps the commonest reason for imbalance and is presumed to be due to a combination of decreased blood supply and neuronal death that occurs to a varying degree as people get older. Usually the symptoms are fairly non-specific and no obvious clinical signs or pathology will be detected.

Transient ischaemic attacks

These are caused by short episodes of brain ischaemia. There are many suggested causes, including spasm and microemboli. The attacks occur without warning, and the patient often forgets what happened. Apart from imbalance there are almost invariably other cerebral ischaemic symptoms, such as difficulty in speaking (dysarthria), blurred vision or weakness of limbs. Unless the attack is prolonged the patient does not fall or black out. If he does the ischaemic episode is not transient and the patient is having a stroke (cerebrovascular accident).

Vertebrobasilar ischaemia

These attacks are occasioned by neck movement, especially hyperextension. The vertebral artery is thereby compressed by an osteophytic spur in an osteo-arthritic cervical spine and transient ischaemia occurs. Disequilibrium is usually the main symptom, but loss of consciousness and other transient neurological deficits can occur. The management is prevention of neck movement either by self-control or a cervical collar.

Epileptic fits

These should present few diagnostic difficulties because of the premonition that an attack is coming, the loss of consciousness and falling with occasional injury or incontinence.

Clinical examination

Because of time constraints it is usual for the clinical examination to be modified to fit a patient's history rather than a full neuro-otological and medical examination being performed in everyone. The following examination is the minimum which should be performed in each individual to identify otological, cardiovascular and neurological disease. It is not designed to identify the actual pathology, but to identify those patients who need referral to a specialist.

Otoscopic examination

This is mainly to exclude chronic otitis media. If detected a fistula test should be performed. The middle ear pressure is changed by applying intermittent pressure on the tragus: if there is erosion of the semicircular canal, in many instances this will result in vertigo.

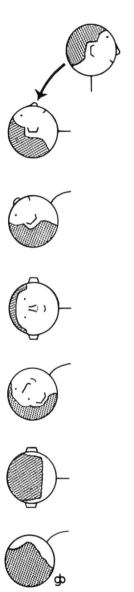

Figure 1.28   Head positions during positional testing. The patient sits on a couch
with the head upright.The clinician then takes hold of the patient's head and having
moved the patient fairly quickly from the upright to the lying position the head is
placed in a variety of positions

Hearing assessment

To identify hearing impairments and in particular unilateral impairments which may be associated with an acoustic neuroma.

Positional testing

To detect positional vertigo *see Figure 1.28*, page 75.

Ophthalmic examination

To identify spontaneous nystagmus. Nystagmus should be assessed by asking the patient to follow with his eyes the examiner's finger moving from a central position to either side (*Figure 1.29*).

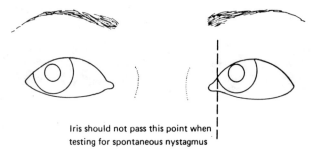

Iris should not pass this point when
testing for spontaneous nystagmus

Figure 1.29   Limit of deviation of the function of the iris, past which the eyes should not pass while testing for nystagmus

Nystagmus is a repetitious slow drift of the eyes in one direction with a rapid correction back to the starting point. If the patient has nystagmus during a quiescent phase the pathology is likely to be central. If present during an acute episode of disequilibrium the problem is most likely otological.

The fundus should be examined to identify papilloedema which suggests increased intracranial pressure.

Cardiovascular system

This is assessed by taking the blood pressure and looking for pulse irregularities.

Nervous system

Specific screening tests are difficult to suggest. The patient's gait should identify incoordination problems of the lower limbs, particularly if he is asked to walk on a straight line. In Romberg's test, the patient stands with his feet together and then closes his eyes. A normal individual should be able to keep his balance. This test can be sharpened by getting the patient to stand heel to toe and/or have his arms raised with the palms up. However, even normal individuals can find this difficult for more than a short period of time.

Who to refer

In the presence of otological, cardiovascular or neurological signs or symptoms it is wise to refer such patients for specialist investigations and management. Radiology, audiometry and vestibulometry may then be helpful in diagnosis.

Management

Having referred all individuals with potential otological, neurological and cardiovascular disease there will remain a large number of individuals with idiopathic disequilibrium and it is their management that is discussed.

As was mentioned earlier, it is important to elucidate the role of drugs by stopping all current medication or changing to a different pharmacological group of drugs when this is unavoidable.

In most, the mainstay of management is reassurance that the problem will almost certainly resolve spontaneously. It is wise to review the patient two or three months later to ensure that this is the case, and if not the patient should be referred.

In a few cases, medication will be necessary for symptomatic relief. Antihistamines, e.g. cinnarizine (Stugeron), phenothiazines, e.g. prochlorperazine (Stemetil) or a vasodilator, e.g. betahistidine (Serc) can all be tried but should not be taken for any extended period because natural resolution of symptoms usually occurs and these drugs can themselves cause disequilibrium.

■ Conclusions

- The diagnosis of the cause of disequilibrium is best gained from the history.
- Drugs are one of the most common and most easily rectified causes of disequilibrium.
- In the majority of individuals the diagnosis will not be clear cut.
- Referral is necessary if there is any suggestion of otological, cardiovascular or neurological disease, in which case specialized investigations may be of some help.
- Otological disequilibrium is worse during the first episode but usually spontaneously resolves because of compensation.
- A unilateral or asymmetric hearing loss should be sought to avoid missing an acoustic neuroma.
- Cerebral ischaemia is, perhaps, the commonest non-otological cause of disequilibrium.
- Compensation with time is normal due to central suppression of faulty input.
- Neurological causes for disequilibrium are comparatively rare and are usually progressive.

Facial palsy

The VII cranial or facial nerve (*Figure 1.30*) leaves the brain stem and enters the internal auditory canal of the temporal bone along with the VIII cranial (auditory) nerve. It continues through the middle ear within a bony canal and then down through the mastoid air cells before it exits into the neck through the stylomastoid foramen which is deep to the tip of the mastoid process. It then divides into several branches while running through the parotid gland, whereafter it supplies the muscles of facial expression.

Within the temporal bone it has three branches, the greater superficial petrosal nerve to the lacrimal glands of the eye, the chorda tympani to the taste buds on the anterior two-thirds of the tongue and the stapedial nerve to the stapedius muscle in the ear.

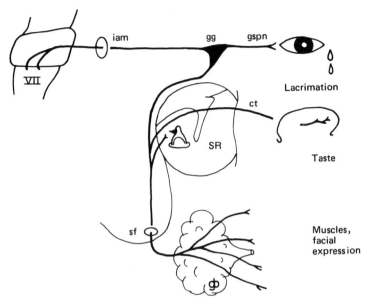

Figure 1.30 *Anatomy of the VII (facial) cranial nerve.* iam, internal auditory meatus; gg, geniculate ganglion; gspn, greater superficial petrosal nerve; ct, chorda tympani; sf, stylomastoid foramen; SR, stapedius reflex

How to arrive at a diagnosis and manage it

The cause of a facial palsy must be presumed to be in the ear until otherwise excluded. It is not that otological causes are the commonest causes of facial palsy (*Table 1.5*), but they are the only ones that can require treatment. In the majority of instances no definite aetiology for the facial palsy is ever identified, but the routine assumption that this is the case inevitably means that many correctable palsies of otological origin are left too late for the outcome to be favourable.

The facial nerve can be affected in any part of its course through the temporal bone, from the internal auditory meatus to the stylomastoid foramen. Perhaps the commonest otological pathology to affect the facial nerve is active chronic otitis media. The inflammation in the middle ear and mastoid can be such that the bone covering the facial nerve is eroded and a palsy results. The patient ought to be asked about an ear discharge, but a negative

Table 1.5 Common sites and causes of facial palsy

Site	Cause
In cerebrum, brain stem	Cerebrovascular accident (stroke)
In the temporal bone	Chronic otitis media
	Acute otitis media
	Herpes
	Head injury with fracture
	Ear surgery
Outside the temporal bone	Malignant parotid neoplasm
Unknown	Idiopathic (Bell's) palsy

response by no means excludes active chronic otitis media as many of these patients do not complain of a discharge. A *competent* otological examination is thus essential and to do this properly all wax and debris must be removed.

Two other common otological causes of a facial palsy, temporal bone fracture and surgical trauma, are relatively easy to identify by taking a history.

If one of the above otological causes is identified an otological opinion must be sought regarding the advisability of surgical exploration, to either repair or decompress the nerve.

The remaining common cause for a palsy within the temporal bone is viral, most often herpes. In a few the diagnosis is obvious because of the presence of herpetic vesicles on the pinna or in the external auditory canal, but in the others the diagnosis is presumptive because of a close time relationship of a generalized viral infection with the onset of the palsy. As opposed to the other otological causes of a facial palsy, the majority of virally induced palsies recover spontaneously and the management is symptomatic, although some clinicians prescribe steroids, which is somewhat controversial.

Clinically, the level of involvement of the facial nerve within the temporal bone can often be identified by testing the various branches of the nerve (*Figure 1.18*). The eye can be tested by measuring tear secretion (Schirmer's test), the branch to the stapedius muscle by provoking a stapedial reflex (tympanometry) and the branch to the tongue by testing taste sensation.

The above, then, are causes of a facial palsy that are quite obviously within the temporal bone. Of the other recognized sites the most common are the brain stem and the cerebrum which may be affected by a cerebrovascular accident (stroke). This diagnosis should be readily made because other cranial or motor nerves will almost invariably be involved (e.g. hemiparesis). When the cause of a facial palsy is above the brain stem, movement of the forehead on the side of the palsy is preserved because of cross-innervation in the brain stem. The other main site for the facial nerve to be affected is once it leaves the skull, the most likely pathology being a malignant parotid tumour, but it is a misconception that malignant tumours will be obvious. Indeed if the neoplasm is in the parotid 'tail' below the angle of the jaw it can be almost impalpable. Benign parotid neoplasms do not cause facial palsies.

After exclusion of the known causes it is normal to call the palsy an idiopathic lower motor neuron or Bell's palsy and this is numerically the largest single group of palsies. Eventually, as a result of research, the aetiology of a proportion will perhaps be found to be viral, another proportion vascular, another proportion autoimmune and so on. In the meantime the main question is how to manage the individuals in whom no aetiological factor has been identified. Various forms of treatment have been advocated, including steroids and vasodilators, but there is little scientific evidence to support their use and they are less favoured than formerly. The majority (approximately 85 per cent) of idiopathic palsies recover completely without treatment. Almost all of the remainder recover to a reasonable extent but an unfortunate few end up with facial distortion which may require attempts at surgical correction. Various electrophysiological tests have been used to try and identify those palsies unlikely to recover but they have not gained universal acceptance because of their variability.

The main disabilities that individuals with an idiopathic facial palsy have are psychological. Once the recognized causes for a palsy have been excluded they can be reassured that it will almost certainly improve. At most any residual weakness will be slight: drooling of food out the corner of the mouth will stop, and the excess eye watering (due to non-draining of tears via the lacrimal duct because of weakness of the orbicularis oculi muscles) will lessen.

The most important complications of facial palsy, whatever its aetiology, are ophthalmological. Conjunctival infection and corneal trauma can occur because of the absence of protective blinking. Partial suturing together of the outer eyelids (tarsorrhaphy) helps to overcome this and should be performed early when complications are anticipated, rather than too late when they have occurred.

■ Conclusions

- Facial palsies should be presumed to be otological in origin until proven otherwise.
- Middle ear infection is the main otological pathology to be excluded.
- The management of this is surgical.
- The other common otological causes are temporal bone fractures and herpes virus infections.
- Various tests of the branches of the facial nerve may help determine the level of involvement within the temporal bone.
- A malignant parotid neoplasm can also cause a facial palsy.
- If no cause for the palsy is identified, it is considered an idiopathic or a Bell's palsy.
- There is no proven medical management for idiopathic palsies.
- In any palsy, eye complications are to be guarded against, especially when the palsy is complete.

The nose

Applied anatomy

The external nose consists of a bony part and a cartilaginous part which are integrated (*Figure 2.1*). The bony part consists of two nasal bones which interdigitate with the frontal bone and the frontal process of the maxilla. The cartilaginous part consists of five separate hyaline cartilages: the septal cartilage divides the nasal cavity in two and supports the paired upper lateral and lower lateral (alar) cartilages.

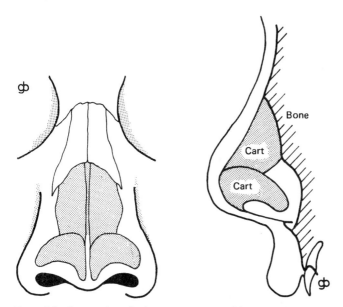

Figure 2.1   Bony and cartilaginous components of the external nose

The function of the nose is to filter, warm and humidify the inspired air and this is achieved mainly by means of the large area of mucus secreting epithelium. Gross particles in the inspired air are caught in the hairs of the nasal vestibule. The air then flows in a well defined manner between the septum and the three turbinates on the lateral wall (*Figure 2.2*). The interior of the nose and sinuses

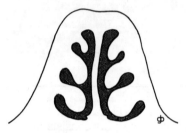

Figure 2.2   Cross section of a nasal cavity. Note normal asymmetric nature of the septum and the unequal size of the turbinates

has a highly vascular mucosa, permanently coated by a layer of mucus which is carried by the mucosal cilia to the nasopharynx where it is either swallowed or spat up according to local culture. This mucus coating warms and humidifies the air as well as filtering out any fine dust particles. Closely integrated with the nasal cavity are the nasal sinuses which for descriptive, but not necessarily for functional, purposes are divided into the maxillary, the ethmoidal group, the frontal and sphenoid sinuses (*Figure 2.3*).

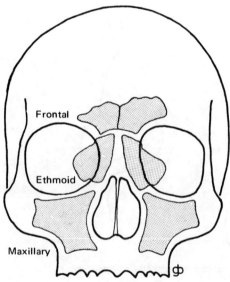

Frontal

Ethmoid

Maxillary

Figure 2.3   Nasal sinuses

These are also lined by a ciliated mucus secreting epithelium and, with the main exception of the sphenoid sinus, drain into the nose below the middle turbinate.

The lacrimal duct, carrying tears from the eyes, drains below the inferior turbinate.

The nose is also the organ of smell, with the olfactory sense organs, situated in the uppermost part of the nasal cavity.

Nasal symptoms

The main nasal symptom attributable to mucosal pathology is excess mucus secretion and nasal obstruction. The nasal cavity need not actually be blocked to cause the sensation of obstruction, an alteration in the normal pattern of air flow is sufficient. As such, anatomical deformities can give the sensation of obstruction although the airway is not physically blocked. Obviously, when in addition the mucosa is oedematous, this will add to the sense of obstruction. Surprisingly, loss of the sense of smell (anosmia) though often present, is rarely complained of. A foul smell (ozoena), due to the anaerobic infection that is sometimes associated with foreign bodies and tumours, can be noticed by others and sometimes by the patient.

Examination

Clinical examination of the nose can be extremely useful in determining pathology: the nose should always be examined externally and internally.

External examination should detect anatomical deformities of the bony and/or cartilaginous skeleton. Internally, anterior rhinoscopy, with the use of a good light and a nasal speculum, should reveal the anterior part of the septum and the inferior turbinate. In some individuals an even larger area can be visualized. There is a tendency to look too high up in the nose and miss pathology on the floor. Anatomical deformities, mucosal oedema and secretions are looked for. Anterior bleeding points especially on Little's area should be definable. Nasal polyps of sufficient size to cause obstructive symptoms can usually be seen, although the inexperienced often consider the turbinates to be polyps. Posterior rhinoscopy using a postnasal mirror is infrequently performed by non-specialists but can be extremely useful in detecting adenoid hypertrophy, postnasal polyps and tumours. If there is any doubt about postnasal pathology an expert opinion should be sought.

Nasal trauma

Trauma can cause damage to either the bony or the cartilaginous components of the nose (*Figure 2.1*), or to both. The bony component usually fractures, while the cartilaginous component most commonly buckles but can also fracture.

A boot, a fist, the 'close stairs' and many more innocent accidents can cause a nasal injury. The mechanism of injury is of interest but usually of minimal help in assessing the degree and type of injury. In the first few hours there will usually be generalized swelling, bruising and tenderness and at this stage clinical assessment can often be misleading. An easier assessment can usually be made 24–48 hours following the injury.

Diagnosis of extent of injury

The first question that arises is 'Has the patient broken his nose?', and here the classic signs of fracture are as applicable to the bony part of the nose as they are to any other bone in the body. There will be swelling and localized tenderness over the fracture line and some loss of function of the nose as an airway. Again, as in all fractures, there may or may not be bony displacement. Non-displaced fractures do not require manipulation, and seldom need splinting. Displaced fractures, on the other hand, do require correction both because of the visual deformity and the distorted airway. The main aim of diagnosis is, therefore, not just to define whether there has been a fracture but also to assess nasal displacement.

Essentially, displaced nasal fractures can be categorized as to whether the main direction of the force has come from the side or has come from the front, though, obviously, combinations can occur depending on how many times, and how, the nose has been hit.

Lateral injuries

Here, the nasal bones are fractured at their junction with the maxillae (*Figure 2.4*) and this is, therefore, the point of maximum tenderness. Displacement, if present, will be away from the side of impact and there may also be nasal broadening. In addition, the

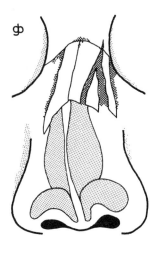

Figure 2.4   Lateral nasal fracture

cartilaginous component will be displaced because of its attachment to the nasal bones. This will be evident by a 'C' or 'S' shaped external deformity with associated internal septal buck-ling. Depending on the amount of septal buckling or dislocation there may be airway obstruction or loss of nasal height. In addition, there may be a septal haematoma which merits surgical intervention in its own right because, if undrained, subsequent infection can occur which can lead to cartilage necrosis and loss of support of the nasal tip.

While it is easy to diagnose a grossly displaced fracture it is more difficult, when dealing with a previously damaged nose, to decide whether the deformity is recent or old. In these instances, reliance must be placed on the localization of tenderness over the fracture site, and if there is doubt as to the diagnosis, little is lost by reviewing the patient 24 hours later. X-rays are notoriously unhelpful in the management of lateral injuries since they may show a fracture but do not indicate whether there is any displacement or airway obstruction which are the criteria for treatment. Radiology is, however, helpful when other facial bones are injured in association with the nasal bones, but it is generally felt unnecessary for legal purposes provided the fact that X-rays were considered unnecessary is recorded.

Frontal injuries

Because of the inherent strength of the attachment of the nasal bones to the frontal and maxillary bones, it usually requires a strong frontal force to cause fracture. Thus, the commonest mechanism of injury is by the face being thrown against a dashboard of a car rather than by a pugilistic fist. Although the attachment of the nasal bones may be firm, the underlying bony complexes, namely the ethmoid bones, the cribriform plate and the floor of the orbit, are often involved because they are thin and, therefore, less resistant.

The clinical feature of a frontal fracture involving only the nasal bones is broadening of the nasal bridge (*Figure 2.5*). It is often difficult to distinguish such a fracture from a pure soft tissue injury due to their similar presentation. The medial palpebral ligaments are, however, attached to the bone and as these can be outwardly

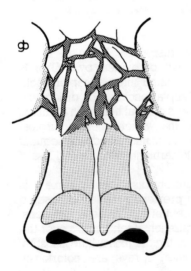

Figure 2.5   Frontal nasal fracture

displaced, measurement of the intercanthal distance may be of benefit, since there are recognized normal values, as there are for the interpupillary distance. Displacement of the lacrimal sac from its groove or direct trauma to the lacrimal duct can, in addition, cause excess eye watering (epiphora).

Where there is sufficient frontal force, the fracture can extend to involve the cribriform plate but this often goes undetected unless made obvious by the presence of cerebrospinal fluid (CSF) rhinorrhoea. This can be difficult to recognize because a runny, bloody nose is not an uncommon symptom after any nasal fracture. The differentiation of CSF from mucus in a bloody discharge can be made by looking for a 'halo sign'. This can be seen by putting some of the secretions on a filter paper. CSF will give a halo of moisture around the blood, which mucus does not. When there is no blood in the secretions glucose can be looked for by laboratory biochemistry or Clinistix, as glucose is present in CSF but not in mucus. Cerebrospinal fluid leaking down the nasopharynx is not always apparent in the anterior nose but is often recognized by the patient complaining of a salty taste in the mouth.

Loss of the sense of smell, although invariably present in cribriform plate fractures, can also occur because the nose is blocked by oedema or blood clots. If the frontal force causing the nasal fracture has a lateral component the fracture line can run through the orbital rim of the maxillary bone, when it can usually be palpated as a 'step' on the orbital margin. On occasions, the inferior rectus muscle may be trapped, limiting upward movement of the eye, and the infra-orbital nerve may also be damaged, causing infra-orbital paraesthesia.

The possibility of the cribriform plate, the ethmoid and the maxillary bone being fractured means that radiology should be performed, although it is often unhelpful due to the thinness of the bones and because the frontal and ethmoidal sinuses will be opaque due to intrasinus bleeding. Tomography can also be helpful but clinical examination is the most important factor.

Treatment

An undisplaced fracture requires no treatment apart from analgesics. A simple displaced fracture requires manipulation within ten days of injury, before reparative callus has become too firm. Under a general anaesthetic, the impacted side of the fracture is outwardly displaced with Walsham's forceps; thereafter the nose is repositioned by digital pressure. In some, disimpaction may be impossible and in these instances there is almost certainly an old fracture which was not previously identified. In these circumstances there is little point in continuing manipulation.

Following a successful manipulation it must be ascertained that the septum has returned to the midline and that any subperichondrial haematoma is evacuated. It is often advisable to stabilize the mobile nose with an external plaster splint and intranasal BIPP (bismuth, iodoform, paraffin paste) packing. As an unsatisfactory result is common, the patient should be reviewed several weeks, and probably also six months, later.

For the patient with an old lateral displacement, the most satisfactory treatment is a septorhinoplasty. Frontal nasal fractures that are associated with ethmoidal or maxillary fractures usually require a combination of closed and open reduction with wiring of the fragments (page 163).

Cerebrospinal fluid rhinorrhoea merits prophylactic antibiotics to prevent ascending meningitis. The majority of leaks cease within ten days but if this does not occur surgical closure via either an extracranial or an intracranial approach, may be merited.

■ Conclusions

- Nasal fractures are mainly diagnosed on clinical grounds.
- The main clinical difficulty is distinguishing between an old and a recent fracture.
- Lateral displacement of the nose is invariably associated with septal displacement.
- Such injuries are treated by closed manipulation within 7–10 days of injury or septorhinoplasty thereafter.
- Nasal broadening of the bony bridge is caused by frontal blows and can be associated with intra-orbital and lacrimal apparatus complications or cerebrospinal fluid rhinorrhoea.
- These injuries are best managed by a combination of closed and open reduction, with bone wiring or packing.

Epistaxis

When a patient presents with blood dripping from his nose the prime aim must be to find whether the bleeding originates anteriorly or posteriorly, as the management of each is totally different. The anterior part of the nose is easy to examine and if an anterior bleeding site cannot be seen the bleeding must be posterior by exclusion. Bilateral bleeding can cause confusion, but it is extremely rare to have bleeding points on both sides. In cases where bilateral epistaxis arises from blood tracking posteriorly around the nasal septum and out from the other nostril, attention should be aimed at the side of the initial bleed.

Anterior bleeding

This is the commoner site but, because in the majority it settles spontaneously, it is less troublesome than posterior bleeding. The bleeding usually comes from septal blood vessels just inside the nasal alae on Little's area (*Figure 2.6*). It has been suggested that

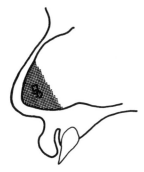

Figure 2.6   Little's area

bleeding occurs from this site because it is the centre of the septal arterial vasculature but this lacks anatomical proof. It is more likely that it is because this is the only area accessible to a picking finger. As such, anterior bleeding is very common in children who often pick their nose unnoticed, especially while asleep. Some adults also have this habit. Anterior bleeding is simple to manage as, apart from the area being accessible to inspection, it can be stopped by manual compression. 'Old wives' consider that ice packs and keys placed on strategic points around the head and neck are of benefit, but wise clinicians do not emulate this. The anterior nose is entirely cartilaginous and it is easily compressed, unlike the bridge of the nose which is bony and non-compressible (*Figure 2.7*). If this does not work, the next thing is to place a piece

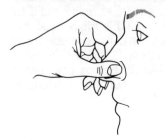

Figure 2.7   Method of compressing nose to control haemorrhage. Note position of fingers

of cotton wool soaked in 1/1000 adrenaline on the affected septum and compress for a further 5 minutes with digital pressure. When the pledget is removed, the anterior part of the nose can be inspected and the bleeding point readily identified. Thereafter there should be no further immediate trouble, especially in children. Their finger nails should be trimmed to prevent any further traumatic nose picking. In addition the blood crusts over the bleeding points should be softened with vaseline to reduce the tendency to further picking. If bleeding continues from an identified point, cautery can be performed using one of the numerous agents (silver nitrate or trichloroacetic acid solutions on a cotton bud; chromic acid or silver nitrate crystals fused by heat to a probe). To prevent damage, the lip or the nares can be wiped with vaseline or the agent may be applied through a metal aural speculum. Packing is usually not necessary for an anterior bleed. If no anterior bleeding point can be identified and the bleeding continues, the bleeding point must be posterior.

Posterior bleeding

This most commonly occurs in patients with non-contractable arteriosclerotic nasal blood vessels. In addition these patients are difficult to manage since the bleeding point is inaccessible to vision and to pressure. In the majority of patients the posterior bleeding point is never identified, but a proper examination should always be performed to exclude any underlying pathology (e.g. neoplasm).

The management of posterior bleeding which does not cease spontaneously is nasal packing. It is only necessary to pack one side of the nose as, at this point, the nasal cavity is bony and pressure on the other will have no effect. The average nasal cavity takes 3 to 4 feet of ½-inch ribbon gauze and this should be lubricated for ease of entry and withdrawal. BIPP or simple vaseline can be used. This packing is inserted in a zig-zag pattern starting at the floor of the nostril and working cranially(*Figure 2.8*). Both ends should be left at the anterior nares lest they prolapse into the postnasal space. This packing should be left in place for at least 24 hours. If despite this there is still bleeding, usually apparent by blood coming down the back of the throat, the nose should be repacked or, alternatively a postnasal pack inserted.

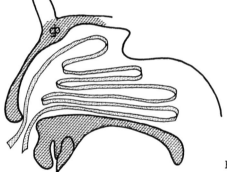

Figure 2.8   Nasal packing

Many methods have been described for this procedure but the most acceptable is to use a 14 or 16 gauge Foley catheter. This is passed along the floor of the nose until it can be seen behind the soft palate. The balloon is then inflated with 5–10 ml of water or air, the aim being to obtain a snug fit in the postnasal space when traction is applied (*Figure 2.9*). The proximal end is then taped to the face and the anterior and middle nose packed with ribbon gauze. The object of the pack is not to exert direct pressure on the bleeding point but rather to seal off the nasal cavity at both ends, by impacting the balloon in the posterior choanae and closing the anterior nares with ribbon gauze. Bleeding is almost certain to stop as the only escape route is into the sinuses which have a finite capacity. Unfortunately, this produces large sinus blood clots which resolve slowly and are, in theory, a good culture medium. It has been recommended that prophylactic antibiotics should be

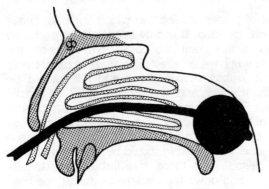

Figure 2.9 Postnasal packing with Foley catheter

given to prevent these clots becoming infected but their necessity is doubtful.

If correctly inserted, a postnasal pack should stop the vast majority of posterior bleeds. In the exceptional patient, surgical intervention may be necessary after several unsatisfactory attempts. As the blood supply to the nose comes mainly from branches of the external carotid artery, this can be ligated in the neck. Alternatively the internal maxillary, which supplies the majority of the posterior nose, can be ligated via a maxillary antrum approach. The ethmoidal arteries, which are branches of the ophthalmic artery and supply the vault of the nose, can be ligated via an inner canthal approach.

General consideration

If there is any doubt about management, patients with a posterior epistaxis must be admitted to hospital and an intravenous drip set up. Blood should be grouped and crossmatched, but it is usually unnecessary to transfuse except when shock is anticipated or where the blood loss is calculated, either from the volume bled or from the drop in haemaglobin level, to be at least 2 pints. Blood transfusion is associated with a mortality of 0.03 per cent.

Investigation of aetiology

Once the bleeding has ceased and the packing is removed, the nose should be inspected for local pathology. Radiology of the sinuses is of minimal value. Hypertension must be excluded after the patient has been allowed to recover and the haemodynamics have returned to normal. Epistaxis is not more common in hypertensive as opposed to normotensive individuals but the opportunity should be taken to identify previously unrecognized hypertension. Epistaxis is common in individuals with a bleeding tendency or leukaemia. In the majority, the diagnosis has already been made because of other symptoms, but the possibility of these diseases should not be forgotten.

■ Conclusions

- After instituting any necessary resuscitative measures the primary aim in an individual with epistaxis is to determine whether bleeding is anterior or posterior in origin.
- Anterior bleeding is more common in children and often caused by picking Little's area on the septum.
- Anterior epistaxis is usually controlled by external nasal pressure.
- Cautery of the bleeding point is sometimes necessary.
- If an anterior bleeding point cannot be identified and the bleeding continues, the bleeding point must be posterior.
- Posterior bleeding is managed by nasal packing. If this fails, a postnasal pack may be required. Rarely, the relevant arterial supply requires ligation.
- In all individuals with epistaxis, nasal pathology, hypertension, bleeding tendencies and leukaemia should be considered as aetiological factors.
- Never underestimate an epistaxis; it can lead to hypovolaemic shock and death.

Blocked nose

The complaint of a blocked nose without any gross symptoms such as rhinorrhoea (runny nose) can be due to a deviated nasal septum, nasal polyps or a nasal tumour. These are readily distinguished by clinical examination.

Deviated nasal septum

A deviated nasal septum is a relatively common finding and the clinician's main difficulty is to decide whether it is actually causing airway obstruction. Complete nasal obstruction can be detected by holding a cold metal spatula below the nares and the absence of steaming up on one side would suggest obstruction. When the septum has been deviated for a considerable period, particularly since childhood, there is usually a natural compensatory shrinking of the turbinate mucosa on the compromized side and a corresponding hypertrophy on the larger side (*Figure 2.10*). This, of course, may not totally overcome the airway problem (*Figure 2.11*).

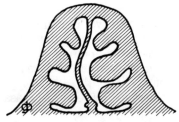 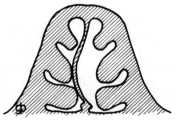

Figure 2.10   Compensated septal deviation

Figure 2.11   Non-compensated septal deviation

If a deviated nasal septum is considered to be the cause of airway obstruction, the only course of management is surgery. This is performed intranasally and consists of either removal of the deviated cartilaginous septum (submucus resection) or, when it is considered necessary to maintain the supportive function of the septum or to correct any coexisting external deformity, then a septoplasty is necessary. A septoplasty removes as little cartilage as is necessary to realign the mobilized septal fragments.

Nasal polyps

Simple nasal polyps are usually bilateral, although they can cause obstructive symptoms predominantly on one side. Nasal polyps arise most commonly from the ethmoidal sinuses, and their aetiology is usually unknown, although they can occur in association with nasal allergy. However, rhinorrhoea is not a common symptom and they do not bleed.

Examination of the nose is usually diagnostic, although the inferior turbinate is sometimes mistaken for a polyp. Differentiation is easy as polyps are insensitive to touch and are mobile.

Surgical avulsion is the usual management, but unfortunately polyps sometimes recur. Repeat avulsion or ethmoidectomy is then usually performed, though some would advocate a topical steroid (beclomethasone) nasal spray. This is sometimes also used as the primary treatment of small polyps.

Nasal tumours

Fortunately nasal tumours are relatively rare but, because of the relative size of the nasal sinuses, can be quite extensive before they present either with nasal obstruction or bleeding. Tumours are usually unilateral, hence unilateral nasal polyps should be viewed with suspicion and certainly biopsied. Sometimes, however, suspicion is only aroused by the appearance of a palatal swelling, diplopia due to orbital cavity involvement or the development of a metastasis in a cervical lymph node.

Nasal tumours are primarily managed by surgery as they are fairly resistant to radiotherapy though this may be given in addition.

■ Conclusions

- Nasal obstruction without any other gross symptoms is usually due to a deviated nasal septum, nasal polyps or a nasal tumour.
- Clinical examination should differentiate these.
- Deviated nasal septa are managed by surgery.
- Bilateral nasal polyps are usually simple and managed by avulsion.
- Unilateral or bleeding nasal polyps should be biopsied to exclude tumour.
- Nasal tumours are usually extensive when they present with nasal obstruction. Extension to the palate, orbit or cervical lymph nodes may be the initial presentation.
- Nasal tumours are primarily treated by surgery.

A runny blocked nose or rhinitis

A runny nose (rhinorrhoea) is caused by excess mucus being produced by an inflamed nasal mucosa. The associated nasal obstruction is due to this excess mucus obstructing an airway already narrowed by oedema. Nasal mucus is clear unless the inflammation has an infective bacterial element, when the secretions will be any shade between yellow, through green to brown. Such purulent discharges are discussed below, the present discussion being concerned with clear rhinorrhoea.

Clear nasal discharge

A runny blocked nose (rhinitis) can be due to anything that causes mucosal inflammation; clinical examination usually confirms the presence of this swollen, oedematous mucosa rather than defining its cause. The aetiological factor or factors usually have to be identified from the history, but laboratory tests and radiology are of minimal value. In taking the history, the most likely cause is often arrived at by a process of exclusion, the recognized factors being viral, bacterial, traumatic, irritant, allergic and non-specific (vasomotor).

How to arrive at a diagnosis

Viral upper respiratory tract infections are the commonest cause of rhinitis but the associated prodromal symptoms, fever and other respiratory tract symptoms such as cough, usually make the diagnosis easy.

Bacterial infections are easily recognized by the yellow, green or brown colour of the rhinorrhoea, seen on examination of the nose either at the anterior nares or in the pharynx.

Possible irritants such as dust, dry atmosphere and cigarette smoke should be considered. Although these are often the only cause of rhinitis, irritants should be assumed to be an additional factor until the other causes have been excluded, either by the history or as a result of treatment.

Nasal symptoms caused by allergy can usually be identified from the history without recourse to diagnostic tests. Naturally, a patient's statement of an allergy needs to be further probed, but it is common for the patient himself to have identified the allergen (provoking agent). This is particularly so when the symptoms are seasonal and can thereby be attributed to factors such as pollens. Such allergies are commonly referred to as 'hay fever' even though hay may have nothing to do with the allergy and there is seldom fever. The allergy is most usually due to pollens from the flowers of grasses, trees or flowers. Allergic symptoms are relatively specific in that as well as the nasal mucosa coming into contact with the allergen, that of the eye is also involved, so that excess watering of the eye (epiphora) is common. In addition sneezing can be marked. In childhood, nasal allergy is found in association with bronchial allergy (asthma) but they are rarely associated in adolescence and adult life. Less clear cut are allergic symptoms due to mites in house dust, animal fur or feathers, but if a definite allergy exists the patient can often relate it to certain situations such as being at home or in bed, with relief when at work or on holiday. After close questioning, symptoms that are not clearly related to a specific factor should not be labelled as allergic without further thought.

Particular care should be exercised in attributing symptoms to house dust mites, especially since many symptom-free individuals react to house dust mites on allergy testing. Allergy tests can be used to confirm the clinical impression of a specific nasal allergy but they are not often helpful as a screening procedure and are often misleading because of the high incidence (20 per cent) of positive reactions in symptom-free individuals.

Allergy tests (*Figure 2.12*) assess the presence of immuno-globulin E (IgE) to various allergens at different locations. IgE is

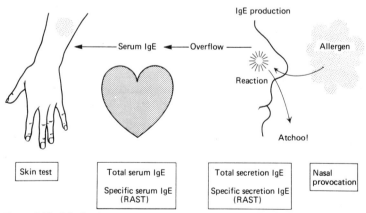

Figure 2.12   Mechanism and investigation of allergic rhinitis

produced by nasal mucosa and induces histamine release and subsequent reactive mucosal inflammation in allergic individuals when contact is made with a specific allergen. The main site of IgE production is the mucosa, so that skin tests only assess whether the immunoglobulin has been absorbed into the general circulation. Serum RAST measurements (RadioAllergo-Absorbent Test) assess the same thing and specific IgE levels can be assessed from nasal secretions (secretion RAST). An alternative test is direct provocation of the nasal mucosa with the suspected allergen but this is not widely used because of the danger of provoking a severe or even fatal allergic reaction.

To summarize, tests should be used to confirm a clinical impression of a specific allergy, rather than as a diagnostic procedure.

If viral and bacterial infections, and traumatic and allergic factors can be excluded, the impressive title of 'vasomotor rhinitis' is often ascribed. There is, however, little evidence to support a vascular aetiology and the title should be regarded as an admission that the aetiology in these cases is unknown.

Treatment of a clear nasal discharge

Irrespective of the aetiology, the treatment of a runny, blocked nose in most cases is supportive rather than curative and the same treatments tend to be given, although evidence for their efficacy has mainly come from patients being treated for seasonal rhinitis. Obviously irritant factors ought to be removed, as should any specific allergen. This is easily done if the allergy is to dog, cat or feather mites but is less easy with pollen or people.

Local steroids   Local steroids such as beclomethasone (Beconase) applied to the nasal mucosa by insufflations are of considerable symptomatic value in allergic rhinitis. Their efficacy in non-specific rhinitis is almost as marked. Systemic steroid absorption does not occur to any degree with normal dosages of beclomethasone.

Sodium cromoglycate (Rhynacrom)   Sodium cromoglycate nasal insufflation is of proven value in allergic rhinitis in about 80 per cent of patients. It is also of symptomatic benefit in a slightly smaller percentage of patients with non-specific rhinitis.

Antihistamines   The main advantage of oral antihistamines against topical nasal preparations is that they can relieve eye watering that is often associated with allergic rhinitis. They are of less symptomatic benefit regarding nasal obstruction. A non-sedative antihistamine is probably preferable.

Vasoconstrictors Ephedrine 0.5 per cent nasal drops BPC or similar drugs may be given for symptomatic relief during an acute episode. Its use should not, however, be prolonged because of habituation and rebound congestion when discontinued.

Desensitization By injecting increasingly larger aliquots of the allergen, an increased tolerance is created in the allergic patient. This treatment is not now to be recommended because of the risk of fatal anaphylactic reactions.

Purulent nasal discharge

Everybody has had a purulent nasal discharge at some time or other and the symptoms probably need little description except to mention that the average patient calls it catarrh and does not differentiate between catarrh that is mucoid and catarrh that is purulent. The clinician always has to make this distinction by enquiring about the colour of the catarrh. A yellow-green or brown nasal discharge is invariably due to a bacterial infection of the mucus secreting, upper respiratory tract mucosa of the nose and nasal sinuses. Such a purulent discharge does not smell particularly offensive. If smell is present and the discharge is unilateral, the diagnosis is most likely a foreign body. When bilateral it is most likely to be atrophic rhinitis.

The common cold virus is the common initiating factor in the production of a purulent nasal discharge. The virus affects a variable amount of the mucosa of the upper respiratory tract which thereby becomes more susceptible to bacterial infection by upper respiratory tract organisms such as *Haemophilus influenzae, Pneumococcus,* streptococci and staphylococci. The mucosa lining the nasal sinuses (maxillary, ethmoid, frontal and sphenoid) is almost invariably involved and contributes to the production of the purulent nasal discharge. Sinus involvement is usually, therefore, asymptomatic. If any symptom is present it is a feeling of fullness of the nose, face or cheeks rather than acute facial pain or headaches.

When facial pain is associated with sinus disease it indicates obstruction of the ostium of the affected sinus by secretions and mucosal oedema. What in effect is then present within a sinus is a non-draining abscess. The presence of facial pain, fever and tenderness over the affected sinus all suggest that this has occurred and this is clinically described as an acute sinusitis, although this term should strictly cover any acute infection of the sinus, whether the ostium is blocked or not. Acute sinusitis is a relatively rare sequela of the common cold or of chronic sinusitis (*see below*).

The purulent nasal discharge associated with a common cold rarely requires antibiotic therapy as the condition spontaneously resolves. Antibiotics are only indicated when there is gross systemic upset or when a specific individual is known to be prone to complications such as acute otitis media. Decongestive nose drops are not usually indicated, but symptomatic relief of any fever is often achieved by the use of aspirin. Steam inhalations encourage drainage of thick secretions and the addition of menthol crystals to the water gives an added sensation of relief.

Chronic sinusitis Chronic sinusitis is the main alternative diagnosis for a purulent nasal discharge. Here the symptoms are the same, with a yellow-green or brown nasal discharge, and occasionally a feeling of facial fullness rather than facial pain or headaches. In contrast to the common cold these symptoms occur frequently and can be unremitting. It is only occasionally that individuals with chronic sinusitis have pain and this usually indicates that the sinus ostium has become blocked, resulting in acute on chronic sinusitis.

When a patient presents with a recurrent purulent nasal discharge it is essential to rule out predisposing factors such as nasal polyps, grossly deviated nasal septum, adenoid hypertrophy, previous nasal surgery and dental disease extending into the maxillary sinus. If found, these usually require surgical correction. If none of these factors are present the individual has idiopathic chronic sinusitis, a condition with considerable similarities to chronic bronchitis regarding aetiology and management. The predisposing factors may be genetic, allergic and environmental, the latter most commonly being smoking and industrial pollution.

There is really no alternative diagnosis to chronic sinusitis in a patient with an anatomically normal nose and recurrent episodes of purulent nasal discharge. Radiology is not particularly helpful, except perhaps to exclude any predisposing pathology. Equally, a maxillary sinus washout will produce mucopus during an active phase and none if the patient is in a quiescent phase of the chronic sinusitis. Sinus washouts used to be the mainstay of treatment before the advent of topical steroids (Beconase) but the latter is now preferred. Septrin, erythromycin, tetracycline and ampicillin can also be prescribed when the symptoms are severe. Nasal decongestants may sometimes be of symptomatic value, along with steam and menthol inhalations. Occasionally, if topical steroids and systemic antibiotics are not effective, the maxillary sinus is explored via a Caldwell Luc approach to remove grossly diseased mucosa or antral polyps but it must be remembered that the maxillary sinus is not the only sinus that can be affected in chronic sinusitis.

■ Conclusions

- When a patient complains of catarrh, it is important to ascertain whether it is mucoid or mucopurulent.
- If mucoid, the diagnosis is rhinitis.
- If mucopurulent, the diagnosis is most likely the common cold or chronic sinusitis.
- Facial pain is uncommon in the common cold or chronic sinusitis and, if due to nasal disease at all, is suggestive of acute sinusitis.

Table 2.1 Commoner causes of rhinitis

Diagnosis	Cause
Mucoid rhinitis	Common cold
	Irritants
	Allergic rhinitis
	Non-specific (vasomotor) rhinitis
Mucopurulent rhinitis	Common cold
	Chronic sinusitis

Mouth and pharynx

Applied anatomy

The mouth and the pharynx are primarily upper alimentary structures, with respiratory tract functions taking a secondary role. Correspondingly, symptoms are related to eating rather than breathing. As well as being involved by local pathology, the mouth and pharynx can be affected by generalized alimentary disease.

Mouth anatomy

The mouth is the area where mastication and primary digestion of the food by saliva takes place. The teeth grind the food and the tongue mixes it up with saliva, which is secreted by the parotid gland opposite the second upper molar tooth and by the submandibular and sublingual glands below the tongue. Food is then formed into a bolus which is propelled backwards by the tongue. The soft palate elevates to close off the nasopharynx and the food enters the pharynx.

Pharynx anatomy

The pharynx is divided into three parts (*Figure 3.1*). The soft palate divides the nasopharynx from the oropharynx and the hypopharynx is the part below the tip of the epiglottis. In the swallowing of food, however, the muscles of the oro- and hypopharynx act as one entity. During swallowing, the tongue musculature pulls up the hyoid bone and, correspondingly, the larynx. This tilts the epiglottis to protect the laryngeal inlet. The food bolus passes under the voluntary control of the pharyngeal musculature via the

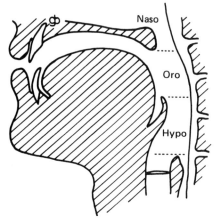

Figure 3.1 The three parts of the pharynx

pyriform fossae into the postcricoid region of the oesophagus at the level of the VI cervical vertebra. Thereafter food propulsion in the oesophagus is an autonomic process. At the entrance to the pharynx there are scattered aggregates of lymphoid tissue, commonly called Waldeyer's ring, which, for anatomical purposes, are grouped (*Figure 3.2*): the adenoids lie in the posterior pharyngeal wall, the tonsils lie between the anterior and posterior pillars of the fauces and the lingual tonsils are at the base of the tongue.

Pain sensation in the mouth is supplied by the V (trigeminal) cranial nerve and in the pharynx by the IX (glossopharyngeal) cranial nerve. Taste on the anterior two-thirds of the tongue is

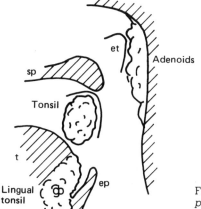

Figure 3.2 *Lymphoid tissue of the pharynx.* ep, epiglottis; et, Eustachian tube; sp, soft palate; t, tongue

supplied by the chorda tympani via the lingual nerve and the posterior one-third by the IX cranial nerve. Tongue movement is controlled by the XII (hypoglossal) cranial nerve and the palate and pharynx by the X (vagus) cranial nerve.

Examination

The mouth and oropharynx can be readily examined provided there is good illumination and a spatula is used to retract the lips, cheeks or tongue. A handheld torch does not give either an adequate light or leave both hands free. Hence a headlight or mirror is preferable.

All areas of the mouth should be examined no matter what the oral complaint, so dentures must *always* be removed. Any lesion should be palpated with a finger. Indeed, if the patient considers there is 'something there', the suspicious area should be palpated even if no lesion can be identified visually.

Examination of the nasopharynx and hypopharynx requires the use of a mirror and as such is not usually within the competence of non-specialists. Correspondingly, if pathology is suspected in either of these areas, referral for clinical examination is mandatory.

Sore throats

A sore throat is a common symptom but its true nature must always be ascertained as patients often use this term when describing other symptoms. Because of the discomfort, a true sore throat should make it difficult to swallow food or fluids and, when severe, even saliva. A feeling of dryness, excess mucus (catarrh), dry cough, altered voice and pain in the neck, are often wrongly described as a 'sore throat'.

A sore throat is caused by inflammation of the pharyngeal mucosa due to either traumatic or infective agents.

Aetiology

Local trauma

Cigarette smoke is one of the commoner causes of a sore throat and the patient need not be a smoker, as buses, cinemas and discotheques usually provide a smoky atmosphere. Indeed, sore throats are common after social events where, in addition to cigarette smoke, the pharynx receives the local trauma of alcohol.

Radiotherapy to the head and neck region almost invariably produces a dry, sore mouth and throat, both by traumatizing the mucosa and by diminishing the secretions of the salivary glands. The effect of radiotherapy is usually temporary.

Upper respiratory tract infections

Viruses, including the common cold and adenoviruses, are the commonest infective cause of a sore throat. They affect a varying proportion of the upper respiratory mucosa, which extends from the anterior nares into the sinuses, back to the nasopharynx, up the

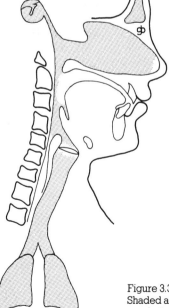

Figure 3.3   Extent of upper respiratory tract mucosa. Shaded area represents distribution of upper respiratory tract, ciliated mucus secreting mucosa

Eustachian tubes to the middle ear, down to the oropharynx and over the tonsils, down the hypopharynx into the larynx, over the vocal cords, down the trachea into the major bronchi and eventually to the bronchioles (*Figure 3.3*). Symptoms of infection of this mucosa vary, therefore, depending on the area that is involved, but there may be any combination of the following: runny nose (coryza), sneezing, runny eyes (due to oedema of the nasolacrimal duct), dullness of hearing (due to retention of middle ear secretions by Eustachian tube oedema), sore throat, hoarse voice and a dry or mucoid cough.

If a patient with a sore throat is fevered this suggests an infective cause, and if, in addition, there are symptoms suggesting that the ear, nose, voice or chest are affected, then the infection is more likely to be viral than bacterial.

Secondary bacterial infection can of course occur, and this is recognized by the watery mucoid secretion becoming mucopurulent. Thus the spit or the nasal or the postnasal discharge becomes yellowy-green.

Following birth, the individual gradually becomes immunocompetent over many years. This requires repeated exposure to viruses and bacteria, the main point of entry being the upper alimentary and respiratory tract mucosa. It is natural, therefore, that in normal children there should be hypertrophy of all the lymph gland tissue in this area. This includes the tonsils, adenoids and cervical lymph nodes. Indeed it could be suggested that in children, non-enlargement of any of these is pathological.

Acute tonsillitis In acute tonsillitis, bacteria, mostly beta-haemolytic streptococci, infect the tonsil, primarily in the tonsillar crypts. Almost invariably there is systemic upset with fever and difficulty in swallowing. The natural course is spontaneous resolution within ten days but this can be shortened to two to three days if an appropriate antibiotic (penicillin) is taken. The infection does not 'go' to the chest, nose or stomach but the cervical lymph nodes draining the area become enlarged and tender.

Quinsy Occasionally an abscess (quinsy) forms in one of the tonsils and this is suspected if the patient finds the mouth difficult to open because of reflex, masseteric muscle spasm (trismus). In the early stages an abscess may be treated with antibiotics but there is the danger of a chronic septic mass resulting because of inadequate dosage. Surgical drainage at that time allows the symptoms to subside rapidly. This can be readily achieved when the abscess is pointing by stab incision under a local anaesthetic.

Otherwise, it may be difficult to find and drain. Tonsillectomy under a general anaesthetic is an alternative under these circumstances. It is considered advisable, if the patient has had trouble with recurrent tonsillitis in the past, that once a quinsy has subsided tonsillectomy should be arranged for a later date. In others it is probably not indicated.

Not all children develop attacks of acute tonsillitis but in those that do the most common age of onset is five to six years. For an individual child, the age of onset may be different but in almost all, natural immunity develops over two to three years and the frequency of attacks then diminishes.

Differential diagnosis of a sore throat

As the majority of children do not smoke, the main difficulty is in differentiating between viral and bacterial infections. Both conditions produce fever and tender lymph glands in the neck. The diagnosis in the acute stage rests, therefore, on the presence or absence of other associated symptoms and the clinical assessment of the extent of the inflammation. Viral infections are usually associated with additional upper respiratory symptoms such as a runny nose, sneezing, watery eyes, cough or hoarse voice, whereas acute tonsillitis is not. In viral infections the majority of the mucosa of the upper respiratory tract will be involved and if any abnormality is detected at all it will be a general hyperaemia and increased irritability of the throat when it is being examined. In many instances no real abnormality will be detected. On the other hand, in acute tonsillitis the inflammation should be obvious and centred around the tonsils which will be swollen, inflamed and oedematous. On occasions 'pus' may be seen coming from a tonsillar crypt but this has to be distinguished from retained food in the crypts. If the diagnosis is acute tonsillitis and the symptoms merit antibiotic therapy, rapid improvement in the signs and symptoms should occur within 24–48 hours. If this does not occur then either the infection is viral or the child did not take the medicine.

In adolescents and adults acute tonsillitis is less common and the diagnosis rests similarly on the above criteria. An additional differential diagnosis in this age group is infectious mononucleosis (glandular fever) in which there is usually lymph node hypertrophy out of all proportion to the extent of inflammation. This hypertrophy need not be confined to the cervical lymph nodes but can also involve any part of the reticuloendothelial system including the liver and spleen.

In all patients, when they do not have a sore throat, clinical examination of the pharynx and tonsils is valueless. This is in contradistinction to the acute situation where it is diagnostic. There is no normal size for tonsils and apparent enlargement is not an indication of past infections so that the diagnosis must be arrived at on the basis of a full history, or by seeing the patient during an acute attack.

When infectious mononucleosis is suspected, the results of a differential white cell count, blood film and monospot tests will be of value. Bacterial culture of pharyngeal or tonsillar swabs has little merit in either the acute or chronic situation as differentiation from the normal commensal flora is virtually impossible. However, in some instances, serial serological tests for viral antibodies may be of value.

Treatment of a sore throat

Treatment is usually supportive until spontaneous resolution occurs, the essence being, especially in children, to ensure that an adequate fluid intake is maintained, taking into account the increased requirements due to fever. Otherwise the patients can eat and drink what they like. In adults, aspirin taken as a gargle and then swallowed, often alleviates the discomfort by having both a topical and systemic effect. In children, aspirin is contraindicated because of the risk of Reye's syndrome (encephalopathy and liver failure). Paracetamol elixir is to be preferred for those under the age of 12 years. In viral infections antibiotics have no part to play unless secondary bacterial infection causes serious consequences, e.g. acute otitis media, and even then their role is in doubt. Antibiotics have no prophylactic role in preventing such complications.

In acute tonsillitis, antibiotics should not be routinely prescribed but they may be of value if the systemic upset is severe. In the presence of repeated attacks of acute tonsillitis, the question will inevitably be raised, most often by the parents, as to whether tonsillectomy would be of value. Fortunes have been made by the adept use of a guillotine to remove tonsils in an attempt to cure all manner of disease. Until recently this has obscured the real indications for tonsillectomy and the attendant dangers. Any controlled clinical trial of tonsillectomy that has been conducted has shown that the benefit is evident for only a couple of years because of the natural tendency for the frequency of attacks to diminish markedly within two years or so. This natural resolution is confirmed in hospitals where there is a long waiting list for tonsillectomy. When eventually admitted the children are usually symptomatically improved and in many the indications for surgery are no longer present. Although low, there is a mortality from surgery which is higher than the mortality from drug reactions to penicillin. The operation is inevitably haemorrhagic and there are psychological problems associated with admission of young children to hospital. The operation is of no value in the treatment of colds, coughs, viral upper respiratory infections or in the prevention of bacterial endocarditis and nephritis. The operation also has a 10 per cent failure rate because of tonsil remnants being left.

It might appear from the above that there are relatively few indications for surgery. It is, however, a balance of judgement regarding the incapacity caused in any particular patient by the recurrent tonsillitis against the disadvantages of surgery. Inevitably the frequency and severity of the attacks must be considered and the balance which is struck will be different for various surgeons, favouring operation when there has been an abscess (quinsy), against it because of the potential of creating speech problems in those with a cleft palate or a bifid uvula, and contraindicated in those with a bleeding tendency. In the absence of palatal problems, this balance is not altered by any clinical finding in the quiescent phase. There is no normal size for tonsils and examination of them is necessary only to ascertain that they are there and to satisfy the parents. This is contrary to the acute situation when examination is extremely helpful in coming to a diagnosis.

It is now recognized that tonsillectomy and adenoidectomy should be considered as two separate operations each having different indications. Adenoidectomy is consequently discussed elsewhere. The tonsils will usually be removed under a general anaesthetic. Guillotine tonsillectomy may still be performed by some surgeons but this does not allow bleeding points to be tied, which is the case with tonsillectomy by dissection.

■ Conclusions

- Viruses are the commonest infective cause of a sore throat.
- Bacterial infections, in the form of acute tonsillitis are correspondingly relatively uncommon.

- Smoking, itself a common cause, helps neither.
- Viral infections are usually associated with nasal or bronchial symptoms (runny, blocked nose, cough, etc.).
- Acute tonsillitis is not associated with nasal or bronchial symptoms.
- Both viral and bacterial infections are associated with fever and lymphadenopathy.
- Clinical examination in the acute stage will readily diagnose tonsillitis as the inflammation will be localized to the tonsils.
- Clinical examination in a quiescent phase is of minimal value in assessing the aetiology of recurrent sore throats.
- A sore throat is managed symptomatically with analgesics and gargles. Antibiotics should not be used routinely.
- Antibiotics have no influence on viral infections but can shorten the course of, but not prevent, acute tonsillitis.
- Recurrent viral infections, colds, runny noses, are not helped by tonsillectomy.
- Recurrent episodes of acute tonsillitis usually stop recurring.
- Tonsillectomy can reduce the frequency of attacks of acute tonsillitis during the two years it takes on average until natural immunity develops.
- A previous quinsy is by no means a definite indication for tonsillectomy.
- Tonsillectomy has a mortality, morbidity and failure rate.

Dysphagia

Technically, the term dysphagia means difficulty in eating rather than difficulty in swallowing so its usage by medical personnel to describe the symptom of difficulty in swallowing is only partially correct and its use should cover the whole range of the problems of eating.

Symptoms

Because of the relative size of the mouth and pharynx, lesions in these regions have to be very gross before there is actual obstruction to the passage of food. Lesions in the mouth and pharynx usually cause the sensation of 'something being there'. Alternatively, there can be difficulty in getting food over but once the food is over there is no further difficulty. This is in contradistinction to diseases of the oesophagus where the lumen is relatively narrow and even small lesions can cause partial obstruction. The symptoms of difficulty in eating and getting it over usually, therefore, arise from diseases of the mouth and pharynx. Difficulty in swallowing usually arises from disease in the oesophagus. In these notes it is with the mouth and the pharynx that we are particularly concerned.

History

In taking the history, it is important to assess the symptoms in detail rather than simply accepting statements such as 'rawness of the throat'. The duration and periodicity of the symptoms are obviously important but their reliability is open to question. It is also unlikely that patients with disease in the mouth and pharynx will have lost much weight unless eating is actually painful, which is uncommon. If there has been loss of weight the systemic effects of disease such as carcinoma should be suspected.

Clinical examination

The clinical examination is the crux of diagnosis in the mouth and oropharynx. In the mouth, radiology has little place except in assessing bony involvement of the mandible or the maxilla. In the pharynx, clinical examination is the single most reliable procedure but when a mirror has to be used, as in viewing the hypopharynx, its reliability is less certain. Where assessment of the hypopharynx is uncertain it is better to perform endoscopy under general or local anaesthesia, rather than rely on radiology. Lateral X-rays of the neck only show up gross mucosal lesions and some foreign bodies, and the main role of a barium swallow is in the diagnosis of muscular incoordination and pharyngeal pouches. The following is a list of areas which if examined during the clinical examination, will allow the clinician to arrive at a diagnosis in the majority of individuals. The list is by no means comprehensive and it is up to the clinician in each individual case to use his judgement to decide whether further areas, such as the abdomen, require examination.

Lips and oral mucosa

Examination of the lips and oral mucosa is the first opportunity to assess the alimentary tract. The lips themselves may be pale suggesting an anaemia, due to iron, folate or vitamin B_{12} deficiency. In these the whole alimentary tract mucosa is affected causing it to be dry and giving a sensation of food sticking. In many who do not wear dentures the mouth may be contracted in circumference and the angles may be cracked – angular cheilitis – due to candidal infection.

Eating may be difficult due to painful, mucosal ulcers (page 159). The commonest causes are recurrent aphthous ulcers and traumatic ulcers from broken teeth or rough, loose fitting dentures. It is usually easy to diagnose candidal fungal infections by their covering whitish membrane which when removed will reveal a raw area. Such infections are more frequent in debilitated patients on antibiotic therapy.

Teeth

Dental problems are the most common cause of difficulty in eating, particularly in the lower socio-economic groups. Thirty-seven per cent of the population over the age of 16 are edentulous and long-term wearing of dentures is associated with atrophy of the maxilla and the mandible, particularly the latter. With advancing years denture fitting and retention becomes a problem and is one of the reasons why a large number do not wear their dentures. Obviously, for them and for those whose dentures are loose or malfitting, eating is more difficult.

In patients with teeth, many of them are often carious and this chronic infection can predispose towards recurrent oropharyngitis. If a large proportion of the teeth have been removed, the normal apposition of the mandible and maxilla is lost, putting strain on the temporomandibular joint. This causes pain in the joint, often complained of as pain in the ear, and difficulty in eating.

The finding of dental problems does not, of course, exclude other pathologies and these must be rigorously sought before attending to the dental problems.

Tongue and sulci

Carcinoma in the tongue is, unfortunately, often of considerable size before being clinically detected. This is because the site of origin is frequently in silent areas such as the bucco-alveolar and the alveolar-glossal sulci. The exclusion of oral carcinoma requires a rigorous inspection of all the areas within the mouth when difficulty in eating is complained of. As mentioned above this necessitates a good light and the use of spatulae so that the cheek and the tongue can be retracted in the various directions to enable the so-called 'silent areas' to be inspected. Finger palpation can also be extremely helpful. Any suspicious area should be biopsied, and particular attention should be paid to hyperkeratotic white plaques (leukoplakia) which often precede a carcinoma. Poor dentition, high alcohol ingestion and smoking are common aetiological factors in oral carcinoma so clinicians should be particularly alert in such patients.

When small, oral carcinomas are usually managed by surgery or radiotherapy and when large by surgery with reconstruction.

Oropharynx

Recurrent pharyngitis is probably the commonest cause of difficulty in eating. In the majority of patients it is of an episodic nature but in some the symptoms can be chronic. In the majority, viral infections are responsible and as viruses affect cell types rather than specific areas the whole of the mucosa of the pharynx is usually involved. During an acute attack of pharyngitis the clinical signs are often minimal. In some there will be a slight increase in redness and in the gag reflex but in others the pharynx may appear entirely normal. When the symptoms are acute, discomfort is fairly predominant. In the chronic situation, this is less so and difficulty in getting food over is more often complained of. Clinical examination in the chronic situation is even more unreliable. Irritant factors, such as smoking or dust, should be identified from the history and avoiding them often improves the symptoms, helping to confirm the clinical diagnosis.

'Big' tonsils are never as big as they might appear clinically, since the act of opening the mouth and saying 'Ah' lifts the soft palate and hence elevates the tonsils into a more prominent position. The tonsils then, although often appearing to occlude the oropharynx, seldom do so and correspondingly rarely cause dysphagia by dint of their size. They will, however, cause dysphagia if they become inflamed.

In the oropharynx the tonsils are the most frequent site for carcinoma. As only one tonsil is usually involved, any degree of asymmetry of tonsil size in someone who complains of 'something there', or food sticking is an indication for biopsy. Histologically, carcinomas are either squamous carcinomas or lymphomas.

Hypopharynx

There are three relatively common pathologies that affect the hypopharynx.

Pharyngeal pouches are relatively rare and are thought to be due to secondary swallow in a megapharynx along with a congenital weakness in the pharyngeal muscle layers through which the mucosa herniates. The hernia gradually extends into the neck and causes a relative obstruction because of external pressure on the pharyngeal wall from food and retained debris within the pouch. As the inlet to the pouch cannot usually be seen either by direct or indirect examination the diagnosis rests on radiological visualization of swallowed barium within the pouch. Pouches are usually surgically excised via the neck or alternatively can be opened into the main lumen by endoscopic diathermy.

Muscular incoordination is an increasingly recognized entity and can be simply local muscular incoordination or part of generalized neurological disease. When part of general disease, such as motor neuron disease or pseudobulbar palsy, there is often overflow into the laryngeal inlet during eating with coughing and aspiration. Local muscular incoordination is akin to inability to squeeze a tube of toothpaste consistently along its length to produce a flow. Muscular incoordination is diagnosed by seeing an abnormal peristaltic pattern on a video tape recording of a barium swallow, and is difficult to manage, there being no specific therapy.

Generalized neurological disease such as motor neuron disease or pseudobulbar palsy is usually much more severe and usually fatal. Indirect laryngoscopy often reveals a lax, immobile pharynx with pooling of saliva in the hypopharynx. Overflow into the larynx and lungs readily occurs with coughing and aspiration pneumonia. Management is extremely disappointing, myotomy and feeding gastrostomy being palliative rather than curative procedures.

Oesophagus

The main symptom that would suggest oesophageal pathology is actual obstruction to swallowing. Pathology most commonly occurs in the upper third in the postcricoid region and in the lower third at the oesophageal gastric junction. Lesions in the lower third are usually the province of the thoracic or gastro-enterological surgeon and are not dealt with here but it is important to remember endoscopy is almost always required to exclude oesophageal malignancy.

Postcricoid lesions have an assocation with iron deficiency anaemia whose mucosal effects have been mentioned earlier and were initially described by ENT surgeons (Paterson and Brown-Kelly). Such anaemias are more common in females and in a certain percentage of them a web develops in the mucosa in the postcricoid region. This causes a holdup of food and actual difficulty in swallowing. In an even smaller proportion of these individuals a postcricoid carcinoma develops. Webs and postcricoid carcinomas do, of course, occur in the absence of anaemia.

Webs are stretched endoscopically and any anaemia treated appropriately. Carcinomas have usually involved the larynx by the time they are diagnosed so pharyngolaryngectomy with reconstruction is the management of choice for cure.

Management

From the above it will be fairly obvious that a clinical examination supplemented by a barium swallow and haematological screen

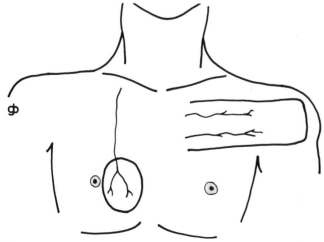

Figure 3.4   A myocutaneous flap of skin is shown on the right and a delto-pectoral flap on the left with their blood supply

will diagnose the majority of pathologies, each of which has its own specific management. In general, small carcinomas are treated with radiotherapy giving a reasonable cure rate, but unfortunately by the time these tumours are diagnosed the majority are large and require fairly extensive surgical excision. The defect that is created requires to be filled by some form of flap (*Figure 3.4*) and the patient is usually given radiotherapy in addition. Disappointingly, the cure rate from such extensive treatment is poor. Currently, chemotherapy does not increase the cure rate but cisplatinum in particular can be of value in palliation. There will remain, however, a number of patients in whom no pathology can be detected. These individuals are often concerned that they may have cancer and once it is ascertained that they do not have cancer they should be reassured. Subsequently their symptoms usually become less pressing. Symptomatic relief can often be achieved by 'moisturizing' mouth washes, gargles or sweets containing glycerine.

Table 3.1. Commoner causes of dysphagia

Mouth	Oropharynx	Hypopharynx
No dentures	Viral pharyngitis	Viral pharyngitis
Dental caries	Tonsillitis	Anaemia
Aphthous ulcers	Carcinoma	Pharyngeal pouch
Anaemia		Muscle incoordination
Carcinoma		Neurological disease
		Carcinoma

■ Conclusions

- Difficulty in eating and the sensation of 'something being there' are symptoms of oral and pharyngeal disease.
- Actual obstruction to swallowing is more likely a symptom of oesophageal disease.
- As part of the alimentary tract mucosa, the oral mucosa often displays generalized disease, of which anaemia is the commonest.

- Clinical examination is the crux of diagnosis in the mouth and oropharynx.
- Dental problems are probably the commonest cause of difficulty in eating.
- Chronic irritation of the pharynx by cigarette smoke and dust is also common.
- Carcinoma should be rigorously sought especially in the relatively blind oral sulci.
- Asymmetry in tonsil size in an adult with symptoms suggests a carcinoma and biopsy is essential.
- Hypopharyngeal disease is often diagnosed radiologically. If a hypopharyngeal tumour is a possibility, direct visualization under anaesthesia is mandatory.
- Pharyngeal pouches cause extrinsic pressure on the pharynx, are diagnosed by barium swallow and are usually surgically excised.
- Muscle incoordination of the pharynx is best diagnosed by assessment of a video recording of a barium swallow.
- Motor neuron disease of the pharynx is invariably fatal due to aspiration pneumonia. Palliation is difficult.

Nasopharynx and adenoids

Adenoid hypertrophy is the most frequent nasopharyngeal problem in children. It cannot be considered a disease as, in childhood, lymphatic tissue is normally active and appears hypertrophied when compared with the adult state. This natural hypertrophy can, however, cause symptoms by blocking off the nasal airway or by affecting Eustachian tube function. Such problems will invariably regress with time as the child's immunocompetence matures and the adenoids reduce in size. In some, however, the symptoms can be so pressing that surgical removal is indicated.

Symptoms of nasal obstruction

Many children appear to have a constantly blocked or runny nose. In most this will be due to recurrent upper respiratory tract infections and the inability of the child to blow his nose. Only in a few will adenoid hypertrophy be the cause and the difficulty is how to distinguish these from the rest. In trying to do so it is surprising how often a child, said to be a constant mouth breather, has no difficulty in breathing through his nose when his mouth is shut. In these patients, mouth breathing is a habit. Inspection of the nose anteriorly should define whether there is gross mucosal oedema and mucopus but this does not clarify whether adenoid hypertrophy is a major factor. If one is fortunate, mirror examination of the postnasal space will help, but in many this is not possible due to lack of cooperation in the child. Lateral soft tissue X-rays of the postnasal space, if performed with the soft palate relaxed, can assess the bulk of the adenoids in relation to the postnasal space. However, in a specific child, it is usually a matter of clinical judgement as to the role of the adenoids in the causation of nasal obstruction.

The other nasal symptom often ascribed to adenoid hypertrophy is snoring. This is a non-fatal complaint but it does give rise to much parental concern. Snoring is most commonly caused by palatal and faucial pillar vibrations during mouth breathing rather than adenoid hypertrophy.

Symptoms of Eustachian tube dysfunction

It has been suggested that adenoid hypertrophy may cause the retention in the middle ear of its mucus either by directly occluding or by preventing the opening of the Eustachian tube, creating the condition of serous otitis media with effusion (page 43). If this retention becomes established, the child may complain of, or be noticed to have, a hearing impairment. This will be of a conductive type because the surface tension of the mucus immobilizes the ossicular chain and the tympanic membrane.

The role of adenoid hypertrophy in otitis media with effusion is by no means proven. Otitis media with effusion certainly occurs secondarily to upper respiratory infections because of mucosal oedema of the Eustachian tube, and also when the Eustachian tube is occluded by a nasopharyngeal tumour. Otitis media with effusion is, however, exceedingly common in children with a cleft palate, in whom the condition is not created by Eustachian tube obstruction but rather by the inability of the Eustachian tube to open because of the defective palatal musculature. A defect of Eustachian tube function has naturally been postulated as a more likely cause of otitis media with effusion than adenoidal obstruction in children. Whatever the answer, there would appear to be a place for adenoidectomy in the management of otitis media with effusion.

Symptoms of palatal dysfunction

Palatal dysfunction can cause two different types of speech defect.

Hyponasality occurs when the nose is unable to function as a resonant chamber when the postnasal space is full of adenoid tissue and the palate cannot relax any further to allow air into the nose. Children with hyponasal speech sound as if they have a constant cold.

Hypernasal speech occurs when the soft palate is unable to close off the postnasal space. As it is necessary to close the palate to pronounce consonants such as k, t, g, d, these sound muffled as they do in a cleft palate child. Hypernasality can occur after adenoidectomy if there is a relative shortness of the soft palate. Understandably then, adenoidectomy is contraindicated in cleft palate children and in those with a submucous cleft, which can be detected by palpating the posterior part of the hard palate.

Treatment of adenoid hypertrophy

If it is decided that the adenoid hypertrophy merits treatment because of the severity of the symptoms, the only available management is adenoidectomy under a general anaesthetic by curetting. Total removal of all adenoid tissue is impossible because of its distribution, so some patchy compensatory hypertrophy of remaining tissue is inevitable. As the indications for adenoidectomy are not the same as for tonsillectomy, there is little logic in performing adenoidectomy routinely along with tonsillectomy unless dual indications are present. Adenoidectomy is not without side effects. Postoperative haemorrhage can lead to death. In addition, the loss of adenoid bulk can cause hypernasal speech especially when there is a short palate or a submucous cleft.

■ Conclusions

- In children the adenoids are normally hypertrophied and in the majority this causes no symptoms.
- This natural adenoid hypertrophy regresses with time.
- Occasionally adenoid hypertrophy may be implicated in nasal obstruction or otitis media with effusion.
- Clinical assessment of adenoid size and extent is often difficult.
- Lateral soft tissue radiology of the postnasal space can be helpful.
- Curettage under general anaesthetic is the usual method of removal
- Adenoidectomy can cause speech problems, due to the development of palatal incompetence and is, therefore, contraindicated in children with a submucous or overt cleft palate.
- Adenoid hypertrophy sufficient to cause symptoms does not occur in teenagers or in adult life. In them a nasopharyngeal tumour is virtually the only diagnosis for a nasopharyngeal swelling.
- Persistent otitis media with effusion in adults suggests a nasopharyngeal tumour.

The larynx

Applied anatomy

The larynx has three main functions.

1. It prevents the entry of food and saliva from the hypopharynx into the respiratory tract.
2. It produces sound vibrations which are modified by palatal, tongue and lip movements to produce speech.
3. It produces coughs.

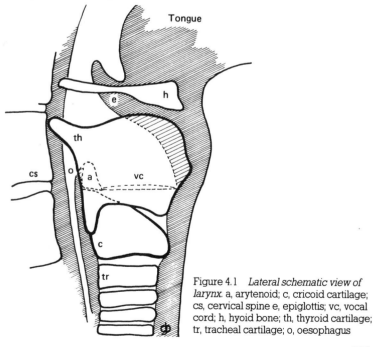

Figure 4.1 *Lateral schematic view of larynx.* a, arytenoid; c, cricoid cartilage; cs, cervical spine e, epiglottis; vc, vocal cord; h, hyoid bone; th, thyroid cartilage; tr, tracheal cartilage; o, oesophagus

It does these by being a muscular structure within an articulating framework of the thyroid, cricoid, arytenoid and epiglottic cartilages (*Figure 4.1*). Functionally, it is divided into three parts as is illustrated in the transverse section of *Figure 4.2*.

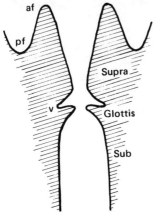

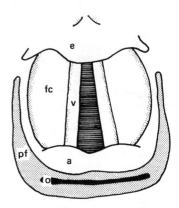

Figure 4.2 *Coronal section through the mid-larynx.* supra, supraglottis; sub, subglottis; af, aryepiglottic fold; pf, pyriform fossa; v, ventricle

Figure 4.3 *Mirror view of larynx.* a, arytenoid; e, epiglottis; fc, false vocal cord; o, oesophagus; pf, pyriform fossa; v, true vocal cord

The vocal cords, or glottis, comprise the middle part and are mainly responsible for the production of sound vibrations and coughs. The false cords, or supraglottis, are above the vocal cords and act as a sphincter to the laryngeal inlet. Their main function is to prevent food and saliva gaining access to the lower respiratory tract and this is done by a combination of its sphincteric action and laryngeal tilting. The latter occurs during swallowing due to the muscular action of the tongue lifting up the hyoid bone which, in turn, tilts the larynx backwards. Normally, then, food goes round the larynx via the pyriform fossa rather than over the epiglottis. The subglottis is the area between the larynx and the trachea but has no specific function.

It is usually possible, with the aid of a mirror, to examine most of the larynx. Behind the base of the tongue will be seen the epiglottis (*Figure 4.3*), from which the aryepiglottic folds run posteriorly to the arytenoids, to form the laryngeal inlet. On either side are the pyriform fossae. Within the larynx it should be possible to see the false and true vocal cords with the exception of their anterior parts which can be hidden by the epiglottis.

The vagus nerve (*Figure 4.4*) is sensory to the larynx and motor to the larynx and pharynx. The sensory supply of the supraglottis is from the internal laryngeal nerve and that of the glottis and subglottis from the recurrent laryngeal nerve. The motor supply to the hypopharynx is mainly from the external laryngeal nerve and that to the supraglottis and glottis from the recurrent laryngeal nerve. Lesions of the recurrent laryngeal nerve, therefore, produce a cord palsy and loss of sensation of the vocal cord on that side. The left side is most commonly affected as that side alone enters the chest and goes below the aortic arch before returning to the larynx.

Hoarseness is primarily a symptom of glottic disease and can be caused by inflammation, neoplasia or a cord palsy. Likewise,

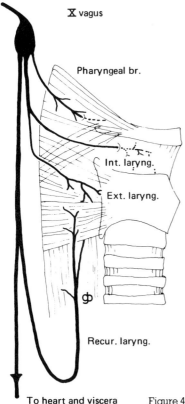

X vagus

Pharyngeal br.

Int. laryng.

Ext. laryng.

Recur. laryng.

To heart and viscera

Figure 4.4   Distribution of vagus nerve to larynx

stridor is usually a symptom of glottic disease. Neoplasia of the supra- and subglottis can cause stridor, but it is usually because it has spread to the glottis rather than that the supra- or subglottis is actually obstructed. Inhalation of food and saliva is a symptom of loss of sensation, muscle weakness or paralysis of the supraglottis which frequently is associated with similar problems of the glottis. Then the problem is, of course, much worse because of the absence of the cough reflex.

Examination of the larynx

Indirect laryngoscopy

The initial examination is made indirectly with a mirror, the soft palate and oropharynx having sometimes to be sprayed with a topical anaesthetic (4 per cent lignocaine) to lessen gagging. This method of examination is difficult and frequently some areas, especially the anterior glottis, cannot be seen because of the epiglottis. As often the main reason for examining the larynx is to exclude a tumour, only experienced clinicians, usually an otolaryngologist, should do this examination.

Fibreoptic laryngoscopy

This technique is particularly valuable to assess the movements of the vocal cords and if the mirror examination has been unsuccessful. The scope is passed through the nose and a topically anaesthetized palate and oropharynx into the hypopharynx from where the larynx can be viewed at rest and during phonation. Unfortunately, as yet, satisfactory biopsies cannot be taken by this method.

Direct laryngoscopy

Under a general anaesthetic the larynx can be viewed directly via a rigid scope and any suspicious areas biopsied but cord movement is more difficult to assess by this method. Microsurgical procedures such as cord stripping are performed via such a scope.

Voice disorders in adults

A voice disorder is a symptom one should never disregard as it could be the presenting symptom of a laryngeal tumour which is the commonest site for a tumour in the head and neck region.

The first thing the clinician has to decide when a patient complains of problems with his voice is whether it is dysphonia or aphonia. Dysphonia is an alteration in the quality of the voice and includes hoarseness. Aphonia is a loss or weakness of the voice. Dysphonia invariably has a pathological basis whereas aphonia is most commonly psychosomatic. Having established that there is hoarseness or a change in the quality of the voice it is important to find out whether it is of recent onset or has been present for longer than two or three weeks as this dictates the management.

Acute hoarseness

Acute laryngitis is something that most individuals will have had at some time or other. It is usually due to the trauma of overusing the voice or tobacco smoke (not necessarily produced by the subject) acting on a laryngeal mucosa whose natural resistance may have been weakened by a viral upper respiratory tract infection. Hoarse voices are, therefore, common after a good party.

Acute laryngitis is usually accompanied by a slight throat discomfort which can be symptomatically relieved by steam inhalations. The inclusion of menthol crystals in the jug of hot water can make it more pleasant but no more efficacious. It should always settle down within a few days; if it does not, it is not acute laryngitis and the patient should be referred for an otolaryngological opinion.

Chronic hoarseness

It is a well founded dictum of medical practice that any adult with hoarseness, even intermittently, for longer than three weeks should be referred. This is not because the majority will have tumours but because non-otolaryngologists are unable to examine the larynx reliably with a mirror to exclude a tumour. Even otolaryngologists do not always find this easy and if they are in doubt they will almost invariably perform a direct examination under anaesthesia.

In taking the history the otolaryngologist will define how much the patient uses his voice, smokes or works in a dusty or otherwise traumatic atmosphere, but this diagnosis rests primarily on the clinical examination. He usually detects one of the following pathologies.

Chronic laryngitis

Chronic laryngitis is the commonest cause of chronic hoarseness. Even if a mirror examination is technically successful, it is often difficult to exclude a neoplasm as they so often arise in a localized, hyperkeratotic area in a chronically inflamed larynx. Otolaryngologists, even if they are fairly confident of a non-malignant diagnosis, will perform a direct laryngoscopy with biopsy in many of these individuals. Once a neoplasm has been excluded, chronic laryngitis is treated by avoidance of traumatizing agents, especially tobacco, and symptomatically relieved by steam inhalations.

Vocal polyps

Benign single polyps on the edge of the vocal cord are not uncommon in adults. Their endoscopic removal is usually effective. In contrast are the more uncommon multiple polyps that occur in children, and present not only with hoarseness but with stridor (page 121) both of which are difficult to treat.

Vocal nodules

Vocal nodules are localized thickenings of the middle third of the the vocal cord, which is the point of maximal contact during vocalization. Hence, vocal nodules are produced by overuse or maluse of the voice and the management is voice rest and instruction in the correct use of the voice by speech therapists. If this conservative management fails, the nodules can be removed utilizing microsurgical techniques.

Laryngeal tumours

Laryngeal tumours are commoner in male smokers and heavy drinkers with rotten teeth, but they can also occur in abstemious spinsters. Direct laryngoscopy under anaesthesia is necessary to assess the extent of the tumour and confirm histologically from a biopsy that it is a tumour, most often a squamous carcinoma.

If the lesion is small the cure rate with radiotherapy is high, with minimal side effects. The larger the tumour, the less effective is radiotherapy, and some form of laryngectomy becomes the management of choice. Laryngectomy can be total or partial, the former requiring a permanent tracheostomy. When surgical excision of the tumour is not compromised, partial laryngectomy is preferable because a mucosally lined fistula or neoglottis can be made between the trachea and the hypopharynx. By closing the tracheal stoma with a finger, expired air will be directed to the mouth to allow the production of comprehensible speech. The more traditional total laryngectomy, which is necessary for larger tumours, is more disabling in that the patient will have to re-learn to speak by regurgitating air from the oesophagus. Not all manage to learn to do this, even with intensive training by a speech therapist. This is certainly one of the situations when it is better to detect a neoplasm when it is small by referring all patients with chronic hoarseness for an opinion.

Vocal cord palsy

Vocal cord palsies can be caused by lesions anywhere along the course of the vagus nerve in the neck and chest and are, therefore, commoner on the left side because of its intrathoracic course. If a cord palsy is detected the clinician's task is to try and determine the aetiology.

Table 4.1 Aetiology of vocal cord palsy

Idiopathic	(?neuropathy)
Tumours:	Chest
	Oesophagus
	Mediastinum
	Base of skull

Tuberculous scarring at lung apex
Arteriosclerotic dilatation or aortic arch
Surgical trauma

The clinician's first task is to excude a neoplasm within the chest and this is done primarily by radiology and sputum cytology. Bronchoscopy and oesophagoscopy may be performed but it is unfortunately rare to be able to cure a chest tumour which is associated with a vocal cord palsy because of the size and position it will have to be before it does so. In the majority palliative therapy is all that can be done. Radiology will also detect tubercular scarring at the lung apex, the disease in most instances being healed and not requiring therapy. Arteriosclerotic dilatation of the aortic cord is again diagnosed by chest radiology. A chest X-ray will help to exclude aortic arteriosclerosis and apical tuberculosis. Another cause of a vocal cord palsy is damage during thyroid gland surgery but this should be obvious from the history and neck scar. Finally, a considerable proportion of individuals will have no obvious aetiology and in them if there are no other symptoms the presumptive cause is a neuropathy.

If a cause for the palsy is identified this is managed appropriately. If no cause is identified the patient is reviewed and in the majority the hoarseness will have resolved due to recovery of the palsy or to compensatory movement of the other cord. Injection of teflon paste into the cord is a simple surgical procedure which can be performed when recovery does not occur and hoarseness persists.

Dysphonia/aphonia

Intermittent weakness or loss of voice without any alteration of the quality of the voice is a psychosomatic disorder. Obviously, the larynx should be examined to exclude any coexistent pathology and if the patient has symptoms at the time of examination he or she should be asked to cough. It is surprising how often a good cough can be produced by someone with 'no voice'. The management is reassurance.

■ Conclusions

- Acute hoarseness is usually due to trauma from excess voice use and tobacco.
- Acute hoarseness should resolve within two to three weeks. If it does not it is chronic hoarseness.
- All individuals with chronic hoarseness require an otolaryngological examination with a mirror.

- Fibreoptic or direct laryngoscopy will be necessary in many to exclude a laryngeal tumour.
- Vocal nodules are managed by voice retraining and rest. Surgical stripping may be necessary.
- Chronic laryngitis is managed by excluding traumatizing factors, mainly tobacco.
- Laryngeal tumours are managed by radiotherapy when small and laryngectomy when large.
- Vocal cord palsies merit investigation to exclude chest neoplasms.

Stridor

The term 'stridor' is classically used for the bovine-like inspiratory noise associated with laryngeal obstruction. This has to be differentiated from a wheeze, as in asthma, which occurs during both inspiration and expiration and is due to narrowing of the bronchioles. It also has to be differentiated from a rattle, which is due to excess secretions in the trachea. The lay term for stridor, especially in children, is croup. Stridor is more common in children than in adults because of the relatively small diameter of their airways, in addition to which the supporting laryngeal cartilages may be soft and collapsible (laryngomalacia) and there may be associated congenital abnormalities such as webs or haemangiomas. In addition, they are more prone to viral infections of the mucociliary lining of the upper respiratory tract (laryngotracheobronchitis). If the reactive oedema is gross, obstruction at the vocal cord level may occur. Lastly, children are more likely to swallow peanuts, coins and other foreign obects which cause stridor either by direct obstruction in the larynx or by compressing the trachea when lodged in the upper oesophagus.

Adults, because of their relatively large airway, infrequently develop obstruction due to infection or foreign bodies but they are more liable to laryngeal tumours, laryngeal trauma and bilateral recurrent laryngeal nerve palsies. The first is because they smoke, the second because they are thrown against sharp edges such as a motor car dashboard and the last because they undergo thyroid surgery.

A group of patients that have to be particularly observed for stridor are those with large laryngeal tumours being treated with radiotherapy as the reactionary oedema to this often initially increases the tumour bulk and narrows even further an already compromised airway.

Diagnosis and management

Unlike most conditions in medicine, diagnosis often has to take second place to management. In all cases, secretions and false teeth are first removed from the mouth and pharynx. This can often greatly relieve symptoms and although it may not eliminate the need for surgery, it can 'buy' time. If there is still an immediate danger to life one of the following must be done, the choice depending on where the emergency occurs and experience.

Laryngotomy

Stick a needle/knife between the cricoid and the thyroid cartilages and keep the hole open (*Figure 4.5*). This is most appropriate for emergencies outside a hospital and for amateur boy scouts.

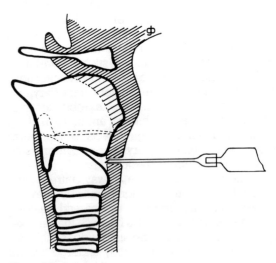

Figure 4.5   Laryngotomy

Pass an endotracheal tube

This is usually the most appropriate treatment in a hospital (*Figure 4.6*), except perhaps following laryngeal trauma or when a tumour is present. It is a skill all clinicians should acquire.

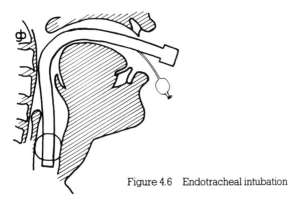

Figure 4.6   Endotracheal intubation

Perform a tracheostomy

This is easier if there already is an endotracheal tube in place, but also essential if laryngotomy or intubation fails.

In a hospital situation both the anaesthetist and the ENT surgeon (or any surgeon that is available) should be called. If the situation is so desperate that the patient cannot wait, perform one of the above manoeuvres, remembering that it is better to have to cope with bleeding and other complications that to fill in a death certificate. If there is more time, the first specialist to arrive will probably wait for the second. Together in a suitably equipped situation (usually an operating theatre) laryngoscopy will be performed to ascertain the pathology. Foreign bodies can be removed with immediate relief. If resolution is likely to occur within days (as in laryngotracheobronchitis, acute epiglottitis and overdoses) endotracheal intubation is all that is necessary. If longer-term intubation is likely, then a tracheostomy is often performed soon after intubation (*Figure 4.7*).

If laryngotomy, intubation or tracheostomy are not performed because life does not appear to be immediately at risk, it must be remembered that the clinical condition can rapidly deteriorate. In this situation it is important to have adequately trained personnel and the appropriate instruments immediately available.

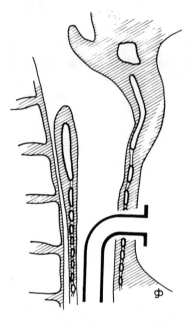

Figure 4.7   Tracheostomy

Once the patient has settled it should be possible to take a history to try and identify the aetiology. *Table 4.2* is a list of the commoner causes of stridor in appropriate order of frequency for infants, children and adults as these are different in each group. It is not usually difficult to come to a diagnosis, the speed of onset and the presence of fever being particularly helpful.

Table 4.2 Commoner causes of stridor

Infants	Laryngomalacia
	Congenital abnormalities
Children	Laryngotracheobronchitis
	Acute epiglottitis
	Foreign body
	Laryngeal papilloma
Adults	Laryngeal neoplasms
	Bilateral vocal cord palsy
	Laryngotracheobronchitis
	Acute epiglottitis
	External trauma
	Laryngeal/tracheal stenosis (following intubation)
	Foreign body

Laryngomalacia

The tracheal cartilages in newborn children are particularly soft. If this is marked the negative pressure of inspiration can cause the trachea to collapse.

Congenital abnormalities

The commonest abnormality is a web joining the anterior vocal cords thus narrowing the airway and immobilizing the cords.

Laryngotracheobronchitis

The child will usually have a preceding history of an upper respiratory tract infection. The majority of such viral infections resolve without severe symptoms developing. In some, perhaps because of a super-added bacterial infection with, for example *Haemophilus influenzae*, the oedema in the subglottic region becomes so gross that the child becomes stridulous. Deaths can occur, so when suspected, hospitalization is merited. During transit to hospital the child should be medically accompanied in case acute obstruction occurs. Thankfully, the majority will settle with aspiration of secretions, humidification and antibiotics, usually amoxycillin. In adults, because of the relative size of the airway, hospitalization is not often required.

Acute epiglottitis

This is potentially a more life-threatening condition than laryngo-tracheobronchitis and is due to a *Haemophilus influenzae* infection of the epiglottitis. This can swell within a few hours and block off the airway causing death. Acute epiglottitis is distinguished from laryngotracheobronchitis in that it is almost invariably associated with pain and drooling of saliva. So if difficulty in breathing develops in a child and is associated with drooling or pain, emergency action is required along the lines suggested for laryngotracheobronchitis, including aspiration, humidification and antibiotics (amoxycillin or ampicillin). In children, examination of the mouth and throat in these circumstances is contraindicated because it can precipitate obstruction.

Though epiglottitis is less common in adults, such an association of symptoms still merits emergency action because death can occur.

Foreign bodies

Here the child is well one minute and stridulous the next. Often this will occur while he is eating but equally what he has inhaled may not be obvious. A back slap is not as good as a quick bear hug around the abdomen (Heimlich manoeuvre). If this is not successful endoscopic removal is necessary.

Laryngeal papilloma

This relatively uncommon condition is akin to warts on the larynx. Warts are slow growing so present as hoarseness which then over a period of months grow to produce breathing difficulties. Management is difficult. Surgical removal by avulsion or perhaps better by laser excision has often to be repeated. Topical preparations such as podophyllin can have a role. Natural resolution will occur over years so until this occurs a speaking tracheostomy may be required.

Laryngeal neoplasia

See page 128.

Bilateral vocal cord palsy

See page 129.

Laryngeal trauma

Mainly because of the legislation which requires the wearing of seat belts, laryngeal trauma from being thrown against a car dashboard with the neck extended is now relatively rare.

■ Conclusions

- Stridor is life-threatening and management often takes precedence over diagnosis.
- The airway should first be cleared of secretions and false teeth.

- Laryngotomy, tracheostomy or endotracheal intubation should be performed sooner rather than later.
- Children are particularly at risk because of the relatively small size of their airways.
- In them acute epiglottitis and laryngotracheobronchitis can be life-threatening.
- The presence of drooling and/or pain usually distinguishes acute epiglottitis from laryngotracheobronchitis.
- In adults acute epiglottitis can also be fatal.
- In the non-emergency situation, humidification and continued aspiration of secretions is beneficial.
- Antibiotics, usually ampicillin, are indicated for acute epiglottitis and laryngotracheobronchitis.
- A bear hug around the abdomen is the emergency treatment for inhaled foreign bodies.

Tracheostomy

Tracheostomy (*Figure 4.8*) can be performed temporarily to relieve upper airway obstruction or to assist lung ventilation. In both instances a tracheostomy tube is mandatory to prevent the tracheostomy from healing over, as it is normally allowed to do once the temporary crisis has resolved. Alternatively, a tracheostomy can be performed for permanent reasons, such as following a laryngectomy. In these instances, when there is no alternative pathway for the air, the tracheostomy does not usually close spontaneously and although a tracheostomy tube is often used, it is not mandatory.

Over the years many different designs and different materials have been used in the manufacture of tracheostomy tubes. At present plastic and silver are the materials most commonly used, the former being disposable while the latter is not, mainly because of its high construction, rather than material, cost. The reason that disposable tubes have not totally replaced silver tubes is that in a permanent situation, there is no need to dispose.

Design features of tracheostomy tubes (*Figure 4.8*)

Cuffed tracheostomy tubes are used most frequently with artificial positive pressure ventilation. The cuff prevents escape of air/gases back out of the trachea during the positive phase of ventilation. The object of the cuff is *not* to prevent the tube falling out – tapes do that. The cuff should only be inflated to the point where it just occludes the tracheal lumen. Inflation to a point greater than this may cause pressure necrosis of the mucosa and perhaps the tracheal cartilage, which almost invariably leads to tracheal stenosis. Fortunately with the introduction of high volume, low pressure cuffs stenosis is less of a problem than formerly.

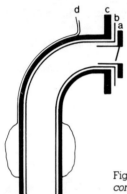

Figure 4.8 *Design features that are available in various combinations on tracheostomy tubes.* a, speaking valve; b, inner tube; c, outer tube; d, inflatable cuff

How then is the correct degree of cuff inflation achieved? It is not by injecting a certain volume of air, as each individual trachea has a different diameter, and it is not by assessing the pressure in the indicator balloon, as the pressure in this does not reflect the pressure within the cuff because of differing elasticity. The correct method is to inflate the cuff until there is no escape of air or gases detected past the cuff and then slowly to deflate it until escape is just detected. The cuff is then at the right pressure, and, unless a one way valve is being used, artery forceps are then applied to the inflation tube prior to removing the syringe and inserting the bung.

Non-cuffed tubes are used when positive pressure ventilation is not being used. If there is no cuff there is no danger of cuff complications.

An introducer aids the insertion of a tracheostomy tube and obviously has to be removed immediately the tube is in place to allow ventilation.

Double tubes have a distinct advantage regarding cleaning. The inner tube is marginally longer than the outer tube and therefore, any crusting of secretions occurs on the inner tube. This can then be removed for cleaning, the outer tube remaining in position in the tracheostome. Single tubes have to be removed in their entirety for cleaning and have to be reinserted, which apart from being tedious, can traumatize the trachea.

Valved tubes are used where the larynx is still *in situ* to allow the patient to speak. Valves are used less frequently than they might be and thereby unnecessary psychological and communication problems are created. Valves are mainly available for silver tubes and are inserted at the opening of the inner tube. The valve is a hinged trapdoor so that inspired air gains easy access but on expiration the valve shuts and the air exits via the larynx, making speech possible. Naturally, a valved tube will not function where there is gross laryngeal obstruction or the larynx has been removed, but the degree of obstruction that will allow relatively easy expiration is often surprising. It is, or course, inspiration rather than expiration that is the main problem in laryngeal obstruction and the tracheostomy overcomes this problem.

Tracheostomy care

In an individual with a tracheostomy the inspired air is no longer humidified and warmed by the upper respiratory passages. The bronchial secretions thereby become excessively thick and sticky and respiratory complications are common unless guarded against.

In the initial stages humidification is vital and is achieved by placing a mask over the tracheostome and moist air is delivered from a nebulizer or water trap. If the tracheostomy is going to be permanent this method of humidification can gradually be discontinued and a laryngectomy bib substituted. This is a foam filled bib which is worn round the neck over the stoma and compensates to some extent for the nose.

The other problem is that the patient is unable to cough up thick mucus secretions so in the initial stages regular aspiration of the secretions with a suction catheter has to be performed. Physiotherapy is also important initially to clear the more peripheral alveoli of secretions. Secretions often build up in the tube and this is where the double tube has its advantages, since it can be cleaned without taking the tube out completely. Single tubes have to be regularly removed for cleaning and, apart from being more time consuming, it is also uncomfortable for the patient.

If a cuffed tracheostomy tube is being used for intermittent positive pressure ventilation, it used to be mandatory to deflate the cuff regularly for 5 minutes to avoid mucosal damage, but with low pressure cuffs this is no longer considered necessary.

■ Conclusions

- A tracheostomy can be performed for a temporary period, most commonly to overcome respiratory difficulties.
- It can also be permanent as when following a laryngectomy. In these cases it is not always necessary to wear a tracheostomy tube.
- Cuffed tracheostomy tubes are used primarily for positive pressure ventilation.
- Double silver tracheostomy tubes have the advantage of easier cleaning and the possibility of utilizing a valve to enable speech production in temporary situations.
- In the period following tracheostomy, humidification, aspiration of secretions and tube toilet are vital to prevent respiratory complications.

How to perform a temporary tracheostomy

1. Preferably first pass an endotracheal tube.
2. Hyperextend neck by placing something beneath the shoulders.
3. Horizontal or vertical skin and subcutaneous tissue incision centred two fingerbreadths below thyroid cartilage and two fingerbreadths above sternal notch.
4. By blunt dissection open a vertical plane in the midline between the strap muscles.
5. Retract strap muscles.
6. If thyroid isthmus is in the way, either retract it or divide between two clamping forceps.

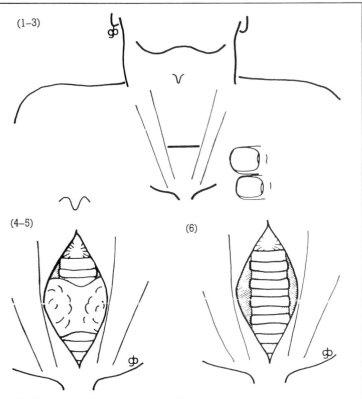

7. Secure hold on trachea with temporary suture.
8. Divide trachea transversely between the second and third *or* third and fourth tracheal cartilages. Alternatively a vertical incision can be made.

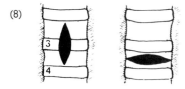

9. Aspirate blood and mucus from trachea.
10. Insert appropriately sized tracheostomy tube.
11. Tie retaining tracheostomy tapes with the neck flexed.

Figure 4.9   How to perform a temporary tracheostomy

Head and neck

Neck lumps

When a patient presents saying he has a lump or swelling in his neck, a long list of potential causes has to be considered to help find out what it is. In the majority of individuals there are always several clues from the history and from the examination of the head and neck which will allow the correct diagnosis to be made without resorting to the attitude that the easiest way to find out what the lump is is to take it out. This attitude is incorrect and, if practised haphazardly, can lead to iatrogenic spread of tumours.

The first thing that the clinician wants to know is where the swelling is. This will tell him the most likely organ or structure involved and thereafter he has to decide what the pathology is in that particular organ or structure. Essentially the lump can be in:

1. the skin and subcutaneous tissues
2. congenital remnants
3. the thyroid gland
4. the salivary glands
5. the bony and cartilagenous structures (larynx, trachea, spine)
6. the blood vessels or
7. the lymph nodes

If it were not for the fact that there are lymph nodes everywhere in the neck, a decision as to what organ or structure is involved would be easier.

Skin

Swellings in the skin and subcutaneous structures such as sebaceous cysts and lipomas should be readily identified by the ability to lift up the mass in the skin. If necessary, these lesions are excised in total and will concern us no further.

Congenital remnants

Thyroglossal and branchial cleft cysts are the two commonest congenital cysts but even these are relatively uncommon. Surprisingly for congenital lesions, they do not usually present until the patient is in the teens or twenties, probably because it is only when they become secondarily infected or when there is haemorrhage into them that they present. Both cysts have classic positions.

Thyroglossal cysts can be anywhere along the line of development of the thyroid between the base of the tongue and the thyroid itself. Occasionally there is an associated fistula, due to the cyst having burst. Treatment is surgical excision of the cyst and its tract.

Branchial cysts, considered an abnormality of fusion of the branchial clefts, are classically situated in the region of the middle third of the sternomastoid muscle (*Figure 5.1*). This also is a fairly common site for an enlarged mid-cervical lymph gland. There is

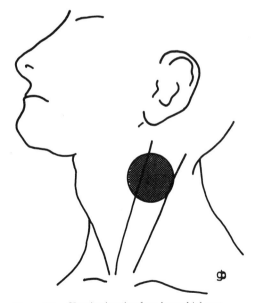

Figure 5.1   Classic situation for a branchial cyst

obviously a differential diagnosis to be made and the factors which have to be considered are discussed below.

Thyroid gland

Swellings of the thyroid gland have a classic position around the trachea, below the thyroid cartilage (*Figure 5.2*). The thyroid is normally attached to the pretracheal fascia and when the trachea and larynx are lifted up by muscle action on the hyoid bone during swallowing, thyroid lumps also move up and this can make them easier to palpate. The relatively rare alternative causes of a swelling in the region of the thyroid gland are pre- and paratracheal lymph nodes, which will also move on swallowing.

Thyroid swellings can affect the whole gland or present as a single nodule. In addition, the patient may be euthyroid, thyrotoxic or hypothyroid (myxoedema). The differentiation between the various thyroid activity states can be made clinically, biochemically or by radioactive iodine uptake. Several clinical combinations can thus result but the initial differentiation is made on what type of swelling is detected.

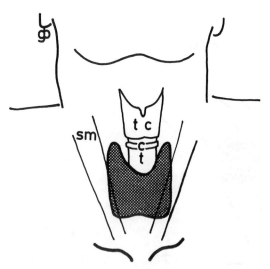

Figure 5.2   *Position of the thyroid gland.* c, cricoid; t, trachea; tc, thyroid cartilage; sm, sternomastoid muscle

Whole gland enlargement

Physiological enlargement in adolescents is not uncommon.

Multinodular goitres are associated with normal thyroid function, the whole gland having a nodular feel though one lobe is often more affected. Surgical excision gives symptomatic relief if the goitre is causing pressure symptoms on the respiratory or alimentary tracts.

Hashimoto's disease The gland is diffusely enlarged secondary to autoimmune thyroiditis which is diagnosed serologically. Thyroxine or surgical excision is the management.

Solitary nodules

The majority of these are caused by benign cysts or adenomas. Some, however, are tumours. Cysts can be diagnosed by ultrasound or needle aspiration. The latter is curative but cytology on the aspirate must be done to exclude a tumour. Needle biopsy of solid lumps should identify those requiring excision to exclude or treat a tumour.

Salivary glands

There are two, main paired salivary glands, the parotid and submandibular, that require consideration. Both have classic positions but, once again, there are lymph nodes in the same position which can cause confusion.

The parotid gland is much more extensive than commonly realized (*Figure 5.7*). The part of the gland that is often forgotten about is below the angle of the jaw, and this can be confused with swellings in the upper cervical (jugulo-digastric) lymph nodes (*Figure 5.5*). Swellings in the remainder of the parotid cause little diagnostic difficulty as to the organ they are in.

The cause of a parotid swelling is relatively easy to decide – inflammatory pathologies cause a painful tender swelling, and, with rare exceptions, all the others are neoplasms (see page 154).

The submandibular gland again has a classic situation, below the middle of the jaw (*Figure 5.3*). Swellings in this region should always be bimanually palpated, with one hand in the submandibular region and a finger of the other hand in the bucco-lingual sulcus. This allows the mass to be better felt and also allows stones within the duct to be identified.

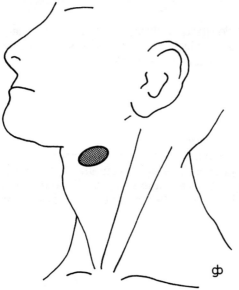

Figure 5.3   Classic position for the submandibular gland

Obstruction of submandibular gland secretions either by stones or 'grit' is its commonest pathology, and a history of an intermittent, painful swelling below the jaw made worse on eating or thinking of eating is classic. Radiology, either straight or with contrast dye injected into the duct, is usually helpful. The treatment is either excision of the stone when it is palpable in the duct or total removal of the submandibular gland. Submandibular salivary gland swellings have to be differentiated from submandibular lymph gland swellings (*Figure 5.5*) but these are relatively rare, except when there is an oral tumour with secondary spread or dental caries with inflammatory lymph gland reaction. A good oral examination is, therefore, mandatory in all patients with a submandibular swelling.

Bone and cartilage

The inexperienced clinician often mistakes the normal bony or cartilaginous structures in the neck for pathological lumps. The most common structure to be confused, especially in thin necks, is the transverse process of the axis which is deep below the angle of the jaw (*Figure 5.4*). The transverse processes are, of course, bilateral but one can be more prominent than the other. Other normal structures such as the hyoid bone, the thyroid and cricoid cartilages should not be difficult to identify. An accessory cervical rib can sometimes be palpable.

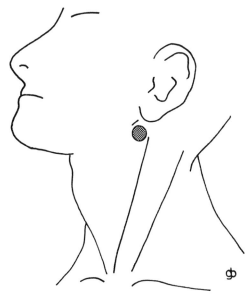

Figure 5.4   Classic position for the transverse process of the axis

Blood vessels

Normally the carotid artery wall is not palpable, although pulsations within it are. Arteriosclerotic thickening of the wall often makes the artery palpable and the pulsations within it less so. A bruit can often be heard by auscultation over an arteriosclerotically narrowed carotid artery, although transmitted bruits from the proximal larger vessels have to be excluded by listening to them as well. Carotid body tumours are extremely rare and do not usually enter into the differential diagnosis of a lump in the neck. They classically present in the region of the carotid bifurcation.

Lymph nodes

There are several hundred lymph nodes on each side of the neck. In adults, lymph nodes are not normally palpable and should be investigated. In children and adolescents it is normal to be able to palpate some lymph glands, mainly because they are chronically inflamed due to the repeated upper respiratory and alimentary tract infections in this age group. Lymph node enlargement in them need not usually arouse too much concern.

The lymph nodes, although generously distributed have a definite pattern of distribution (*Figure 5.5*), the only groups which are inaccessible to palpation being the retropharyngeal nodes. Their pattern of drainage from the different areas of the head and neck is also relatively constant (*Figure 5.6*), although in any disease process not all nodes in the chain draining the affected part are necessarily affected. Thus, an inflammatory lesion at the tip of the tongue may involve only a lower cervical lymph node.

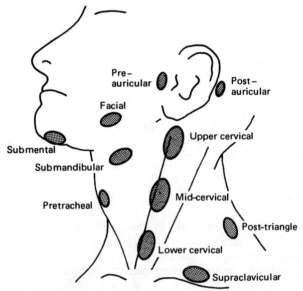

Figure 5.5   Classic pattern of distribution of neck lymph nodes

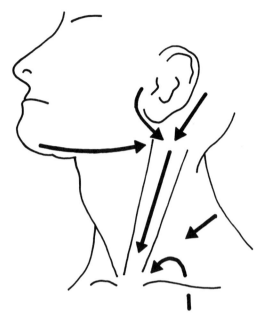

Figure 5.6   Pattern of drainage of neck lymph nodes

If a lymph node is enlarged it implies pathology in the head and neck region, the only exception being the supraclavicular nodes. These nodes also drain from the thorax and, in addition, on the left there is drainage from the upper abdomen because of the relationship to the thoracic duct. The function of the lymph nodes, as anywhere in the body, is to provide a local defence mechanism against inflammation of any type, most commonly infective or neoplastic. The clinician's task is usually to differentiate between these and to define the primary site of the infection or neoplasm.

Lymph node enlargement due to infection

Lymph node enlargements which are secondary to inflammation are, or at some time have been, painful. Often several glands are affected and they usually are, or at some stage have been, tender to palpation. The most common sites to be infected are the teeth, nose and pharynx. Correspondingly, the upper cervical (jugulo-digastric) lymph glands are the ones most commonly affected. As stated earlier, palpable lymph nodes are common in children, who normally have recurrent upper respiratory and oropharyngeal infections.

In adolescents, infectious mononucleosis must be considered. Here the lymphadenopathy is usually multiple and bilateral and can involve lymph gland groups apart from those of the head and neck.

In adults infective enlargement of a lymph node is uncommon and neoplasm is the more likely possibility. Primary tuberculosis of the neck nodes is however still a possibility following ingestion of the organisms and is not necessarily associated with pulmonary tuberculosis. Recent immigrants from the developing nations are particularly at risk and as the infection is chronic, the nodes are not usually tender. Occasionally, cervical tuberculosis may present as an abscess or as a fistula, but more often the diagnosis is arrived at histologically when the node is excised to exclude a neoplasm.

Lymph node enlargement due to neoplasm

In adults, an enlarged lymph node in the neck must be considered a neoplasm until proven otherwise. In adults under the age of 40, the most likely neoplasm is a lymphoma. In those over 40, it is likely to be a secondary from a primary squamous carcinoma from somewhere in the head and neck.

In all patients the first thing to do is to examine thoroughly the head and neck, paying particular attention to other lymphatic tissue in the tonsils, the postnasal space and the base of the tongue. The area which primarily drains to the enlarged node should be examined but not to the exclusion of the other areas. The primary site for a squamous carcinoma is very often silent, that is without symptoms or signs. This is not surprising as the head and neck have many spaces where a neoplasm has to be fairly big before it causes symptoms. Examples of such spaces are the nasopharynx, the pyriform fossae, the supraglottis, the base of tongue, the tonsil and the oral cavity, The majority of these sites are not easy to examine and it should, therefore, be the rule that an otolaryngologist should examine every adult with a neck swelling. Having completed the examination, the otolaryngologist will be faced with one of two situations which are handled in different ways.

1. *Obvious primary with secondary lymph node involvement.* Endoscopy to assess the extent of the tumour along with biopsy to confirm the diagnosis will be carried out but the neck node will not be biopsied, as the reason for its enlargement is obvious

and biopsy has the risk of disseminating the tumour to the skin. A pathological diagnosis of squamous carcinoma having been achieved, the primary and secondary tumours are surgically removed *en bloc*, as this gives the best chance of cure.

2. **Node(s) with no obvious primary.** Endoscopy under a general anaesthetic of the entire upper alimentary and respiratory tract will be carried out in search of a small primary such as in the postnasal space. If none is identified, needle biopsy or excision biopsy of the node is carried out. If a squamous carcinoma is identified block neck dissection, to cure the obvious tumour, and radiotherapy to the head and neck, to treat what is assumed to be an occult primary, is given. If a lymphoma is identified, the liver, spleen, abdominal lymph nodes and the marrow are assessed to stage the tumour. Radiotherapy is usually given to disease localized in the head and neck and chemotherapy given for generalized disease. If only non-specific reactive changes are histologically present and there is no obvious source for the inflammation, for example in the teeth, nothing further is done.

The otolaryngologist himself will normally not be happy to exclude a primary neoplasm without performing a direct examination of all these areas under a general anaesthetic.

It is generally considered better to biopsy the primary site rather than the secondarily involved lymph node as this can lead to further local spread. When there are multiple lymph node enlargements, either on one or both sides of the neck, the neoplasm is often one of the reticuloses, for example Hodgkin's disease.

■ Conclusions

- Neck masses can be in the skin, congenital remnants, the thyroid or salivary glands, the bony or cartilaginous structures or the lymph nodes.
- The site of the mass will usually distinguish the tissue of origin.
- The age of the patient, the history and a full ENT examination will usually distinguish between the various pathologies.
- Lymph nodes are the commonest neck masses.

- Inflammatory nodes usually are or have been tender.
- Palpable lymph nodes in children are normal.
- Palpable lymph nodes in adults, unless residual from childhood, are definitely pathological.
- In an adult over 40 years of age, the cause of enlargement of a neck lymph node is most commonly neoplasm in the head and neck. A competent and thorough ENT examination is, therefore, required.

Parotid swellings

Swellings in the area of the parotid gland (*Figure 5.7(a)*) are often not as easy to diagnose and identify as one might hope. Parotid swellings are often only intermittently present and they can be confused with lymph glands, both in front of the ear and over the facial vessels (*Figure 5.5*, page 148). It must also be remembered

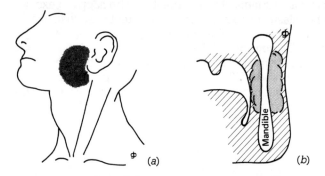

Figure 5.7 (a)   Normal anatomical position of the parotid gland. (b)   Location of the parotid around mandible

that the tail of the parotid extends below the angle of the jaw so that parotid pathology can present as a 'lump' in the neck. The parotid also extends medial to the masseter and buccinator muscles and can present as an intra-oral swelling in the region of the tonsils (*Figure 5.7(b)*). To reach a diagnosis the usual clinical history and examination will be performed. These can be of help, but in coming to a pathological diagnosis the main consideration will be whether the swelling is acute, intermittent or chronic. In addition, whether the swelling is painful or tender to touch and whether the swelling is unilateral or bilateral is helpful (*Table 5.1*).

Table 5.1

Parotid swellings	Pain/tenderness	Bilateral
Acute		
Mumps	x	x
Bacterial parotitis	x	–
Intermittent		
Stones	x	–
Autoimmune disease	x	x
Chronic		
Tumours	–	–

Acute swellings

These are the easiest to diagnose and are usually due to either bacterial or viral infections causing an *acute parotitis*.

Bacterial parotitis can occur if the salivary flow diminishes thereby making it easier for the normal bacterial flora to ascend the parotid duct to cause infection. Before the necessity for adequate fluid replacement in severely ill patients was recognized, this used to occur frequently in debilitated patients but is fortunately now uncommon.

Mumps is the commonest virus aetiology, easily identified by its bilateral occurrence and perhaps by the dreaded complication of orchitis, pancreatitis or deafness. In both bacterial and viral infections the patient will be ill, pyrexial and the parotid will be tender to palpation. The distinction is usually easy, mumps being more often bilateral and in children and not usually having pus exuding from the parotid duct. Therapy in bacterial parotitis is rehydration, antibiotics and incision drainage if abscess formation has occurred. Mumps is treated expectantly and hopefully prevented by immunization.

Intermittent swellings

By this is meant periodic enlargement of the parotid gland which may or may not reduce to a normal size in between. Normally the gland is impalpable.

Stones

These rarely cause parotid swellings but are suggested when the swelling is associated with preprandial distension or discomfort. Parotid swellings associated with stones frequently last for days which is in contrast to submandibular swellings which resolve within hours. The stone can usually be palpated unless it is embedded in the gland, from which it may be milked by manual palpation. In the parotid, small particles of 'grit' more commonly cause intermittent swelling but, because they are impalpable, they are diagnosed by sialography. Radio-opaque dye is injected through a cannula into the parotid duct which outlines the ducts and readily identifies any obstruction. If there has been an associated intermittent low grade infection there may be fibrotic narrowing of the ducts with distal dilatation; *sialectasis.* The treatment of stones is surgical removal. Swellings due to grit particles usually improve following radiology because this has washed them out.

Autoimmune disease

These cause intermittent, bilateral parotid enlargement, most often in middle aged women. There can be manifestations of other autoimmune diseases and certain combinations have been given syndrome titles. The commonest is Sjögren's syndrome, which is a triad of intermittent parotid swelling associated with dry eyes (keratoconjunctivitis) and rheumatoid arthritis. The volume of lacrimation is reduced when measured by Shirmer's test, in which the tears are absorbed by a strip of filter or litmus paper hooked into the inferior fornix of the eye. The condition is usually progressive with the decreased salivary secretion producing a dry mouth (xerostomia) and gross dental caries in the dentulous patient. As in all autoimmune disorders, progression to lymphoma can occur. The diagnosis is confirmed by serology.

If neoplasia can be excluded treatment is expectant, steroids having a minimal part to play. If there is doubt about the diagnosis or if symptoms are severe, parotidectomy can be performed.

Persistent swellings

A persistent unilateral parotid swelling is almost certainly a tumour, most frequently however, being benign. Unless there is a facial palsy, skin ulceration or grossly enlarged cervical lymph nodes it is difficult to determine clinically which parotid tumours are malignant. The majority of both benign and malignant tumours are pain free. In the majority the initial management is superficial parotidectomy rather than biopsy or enucleation and this will cure a benign tumour. If malignancy is then detected histologically, total parotidectomy with sacrifice of the facial nerve is usually performed as radiotherapy has little part to play in most parotid tumours.

■ Conclusions

- Bilateral acute parotid swellings are most commonly due to mumps.
- A unilateral, acute parotid swelling is most likely due to acute parotitis.
- Intermittent parotid swellings can be due to either autoimmune disease, duct stones or grit.
- Persistent parotid swellings are tumours. They are usually painless and, because the majority are benign, superficial parotidectomy is diagnostic and curative for most of them.

Pain in the head and neck

Facial pain is a symptom that clinicians often find more difficult to diagnose than should be the case. A large proportion of individuals with facial pain do not have any identifiable pathology and the clinician often feels he has to ascribe an unjustifiable title such as sinusitis or eye strain. This can cause considerable confusion and mismanagement but the problem can be logically managed by taking a good history and by thoroughly examining the ear, nose and mouth. The causal pathology, if any, will then in most instances be identified without recourse to investigations.

Pain in the head and neck can originate in any of the head and neck structures, but these are all supplied by one of two nerves. The V cranial nerve is sensory to the skin of the face, neck and ear, to the mucosa of the nose, sinuses and oral cavity and anterior two-thirds of the tongue and to the teeth (*Figure 5.8*). The IX cranial

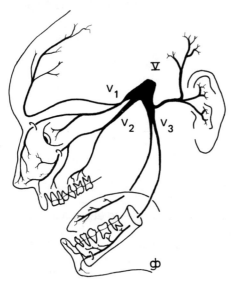

Figure 5.8   Sensory distribution of the three branches (V_1, V_2, V_3) of the V (trigeminal) cranial nerve

nerve is sensory to the pharynx (naso-, oro- and hypopharynx), posterior one-third of the tongue, Eustachian tube and middle ear (*Figure 5.9*). Pain can be either localized to the site of the disease or can be referred. When trying to identify the pathology one must, therefore, look first where the patient complains of the pain. If there is local disease there will usually be signs of inflammation and tenderness to touch. If no pathology is detected, then the clinician must examine elsewhere to exclude the causes of referred pain. Thus, if pain is complained of in the ear, the ear is first examined and if no local pathology is detected the areas of distribution of both the V and IX cranial nerves, from which the ear receives a sensory supply have to be examined. Referred pain is probably as common, if not commoner, than locally produced pain. The following is a discussion of head and neck diseases which can

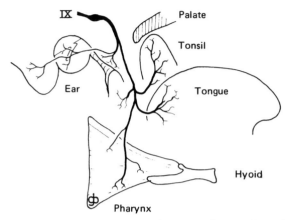

Figure 5.9   Sensory distribution of IX (glossopharyngeal) cranial nerve

cause pain and they will be considered primarily as causing local pain but it must be remembered that they all can present as pain elsewhere in the head and neck.

Earache (otalgia) (*see also* page 28)

Local causes

There are two external auditory canal conditions that commonly cause pain – otitis externa and boils. In both, the canal will be oedematous and narrow, and pressing the tragus will elicit tenderness.

Middle ear pathologies cause pain by exerting either a positive or negative pressure on an intact tympanic membrane. *Acute otitis media,* which is primarily a bacterial infection of the middle ear, causes acute pain as long as the tympanic membrane is intact but subsides with rupture of the tympanic membrane and the release of pus. Otitis media with effusion is a non-bacterial process and is by no means invariably associated with earache, but when it occurs it is due to the negative pressure in the middle ear.

Pain is infrequent in chronic otitis media because the permanent tympanic membrane perforation allows any mucopus to drain and there is, therefore, no build up of pressure. Occasionally, however, blockage of infected material in the mastoid aircell system occurs and *acute mastoiditis* develops. Here there will be tenderness

158

over the mastoid bone. Alternatively, if the infection spreads to the dura, causing meningitis or an intracranial abscess, the earliest symptom is usually headache. The clinical finding here is nuchal discomfort and rigidity on flexion of the neck.

Although not strictly otological, the *temporomandibular* joint is in such close relation to the ear that inflammatory disease of the joint often presents as otolgia. The tenderness is anterior to the external auditory canal and pain is made worse on movement of the jaw or straining against resistance. The commonest cause of temporomandibular joint pain is the non-wearing of, or badly fitting, dentures which allow the jaw to move in a random, ill-defined manner which puts strain on the joint.

Referred causes

Dental caries, oropharyngeal inflammation and cervical osteoarthritis are the commonest causes of referred otalgia. In the absence of otological or temporomandibular joint disease, the mouth, throat and neck must be examined. Dental caries should be obvious by inspecting the cusps of the teeth and looking at the dental–alveolar junctions (*Figure 5.10*). Oropharyngeal lesions

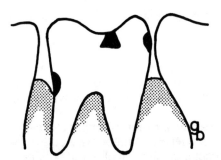

Figure 5.10   Commoner sites for dental caries

and, in particular, tumours will be looked for. A diagnostic problem that frequently presents in children is whether otalgia is due to an upper respiratory tract infection with a mild oropharyngitis or due to acute otitis media with effusion. As these are frequently associated with an upper respiratory infection the crux of the diagnosis rests on the otoscopic appearance of either inflammation or retraction. Cervical osteoarthritis can usually be diagnosed if gently, but fully, moving the neck in all directions, including rotating, causes pain. The management is advice on neck movements and a cervical collar when particularly troublesome.

Sore or painful mouth

Local causes

Small mucosal ulcers are usually painful and the diagnosis is made from experience and their site.

Aphthous ulcers recur regularly on mobile parts of the mucosa such as the cheek and labiogingival sulci. Their treatment is topical antiseptics (chlorhexidine), astringents (zinc sulphate BPC) or hydrocortisone pellets.

Traumatic ulcers from jagged teeth or dentures are usually identified as such by the patient or by the clinician looking for a cause. Dental management is curative.

Candida yeast infections are covered by a white membrane which when removed reveals a raw mucosal area. These areas are often under the upper dentures and patients may also have a small painful mouth with cracks at the angles: *angular cheilitis*. Patients with candidal infection are often debilitated by generalized disease and have been on antibiotic therapy. Treatment is with topical nystatin lozenges, cessation of antibiotics and by improved general health.

Herpetic ulcers occur on non-mobile mucosa such as the hard palate and are treated non-specifically with protective pastes (carmellose gelatin: Orabase).

Sore or painful throat

Local causes

By common usage a 'sore' throat is a slightly different symptom from pain in the throat. When the act of swallowing causes particular discomfort it is usually described as a sore throat and when there is no particular relationship to swallowing it is called a pain. Viral pharyngitis and bacterial tonsillitis are the commonest causes of sore throat but trauma from cigarette smoke and excessive voice usage should not be forgotten. In the majority of individuals the findings are non-specific because of the wide variation of normal appearance of the pharynx. The throat, however, will be tender and a marked gag reflex is common. In acute tonsillitis there will usually be pus exuding from the crypts and in many the mouth will be slightly difficult to open because of protective spasm of the masticatory muscles.

Local causes of pain in the throat are relatively uncommon but glossopharyngeal neuralgia and invasive neoplasms should not be forgotten.

Referred pain

Angina pectoris and, more rarely, cervical osteoarthritis are the commoner causes of referred pain to the throat.

Toothache

Local causes

Dental caries are so common that it is rare, except in edentulous patients, not to be able to suggest that they have some part to play in a patient with facial pain. Dental caries are usually fairly obvious when they affect the crowns of the teeth, but they are also exceptionally common between the teeth and at the junction with the gums and this is more difficult to identify (*Figure 5.10*). Dental root abscesses are, of course, a cause of severe toothache, and here local tenderness will be pronounced and a palpable swelling of the maxilla or the jaw may be evident. The best test is to tap the appropriate tooth, which will cause discomfort.

Referred pain

Referred pain to the teeth is mainly from the maxillary sinus but, because of the close anatomical proximity, it could well be that in many it is actual maxillary sinus disease involving the teeth.

Frontal headache

Local causes

Frontal headaches are extremely common but sinusitis is a rare cause of such a headache. The vast majority of individuals with frontal headache have no definable cause. Chronic sinusitis is invariably associated with nasal discharge: a patient without a clear cut relationship between frontal headaches and nasal discharge is unlikely to be suffering from sinusitis. Acute frontal sinusitis is rare but it can cause acute rather than recurrent or chronic frontal pain. Here there is invariably tenderness over the frontal sinus.

Temporal arteritis is an even rarer cause of frontal headaches and here a tender thickened arterial wall in the temple region may be palpated.

Referred pain

This is rare to the frontal region. The majority of patients with frontal headache have no definable aetiology.

Pain between the eyes and over the cheeks

Local causes

In the majority of individuals with pain between the eyes and over the cheeks neither a local nor a referred cause can be identified. Idiopathic pain is, therefore, the commonest diagnosis but should only be ascribed once the recognized causes have been excluded.

The ethmoid and maxillary sinuses, when affected by acute sinusitis, cause severe local discomfort, readily identified by tenderness on local pressure and perhaps secondary soft tissue oedema of the overlying tissues. Mucopus will usually be evident in the nose. Chronic sinusitis can cause pain in these areas but it is extremely rare to have chronic sinusitis without mucopurulent rhinorrhoea and without clinical evidence of infection in the nose.

Ophthalmological causes of facial pain are uncommon, although eye tests are often recommended. Uncorrected errors of refraction can cause discomfort but should only be diagnosed if it is brought about by prolonged use of the eyes in otherwise poor visual circumstances such as poor lighting.

Trigeminal neuralgia is usually diagnosed by its episodic occurrence, its severity, its area of distribution of the trigeminal nerve, the presence of triggering factors such as eating and by its dramatic response to carbamazepine (Tegretol).

Referred pain

This is uncommon in this area, except for angina pectoris.

Pains in the nose

Local causes

Boils of the skin in the vestibule of the nose cause acute pain but are readily identifiable.

Some individuals complain of a sensation of burning or discomfort in the nose, but without any locally identifiable pathology. It would be reasonable to assume a local traumatic factor in these cases and to advise accordingly.

Referred pain

This is uncommon in the nose.

Occipital headache

Local causes

Cervical osteoarthritis is extremely common and can cause pain either on movement of the neck or because of the secondary muscular spasm. Clinical examination of the neck should detect osteoarthritis by the lack of movement and also by triggering of the discomfort which, on occasions, may radiate down the arm. Radiology is of minimal value as the majority of normal adults will have some evidence of cervical osteoarthritis, whether or not this is causing symptoms.

Referred pain

This is uncommon.

Pain in the neck

Local causes

Inflamed cervical lymph glands are the commonest cause of pain, and the glands will be palpable and tender. Occasionally, a neck abscess can develop from a lymph gland. These will all be secondary to infection elsewhere in the head and neck and the site of origin should be carefully looked for.

Pharyngitis and laryngitis, most often viral in origin, may be felt mainly as a discomfort in the neck rather than the throat. Here there will be tenderness on palpation of the pharynx or larynx which is made worse on movement of these structures.

Referred pain

This is uncommon in the neck.

■ Conclusions

- Facial pain is often idiopathic, but local and referred causes of pain must be excluded.
- Otalgia is more often referred rather than locally derived pain.
- Sinusitis without nasal symptoms or signs is an extremely rare cause of facial pain.
- Facial pain is rarely caused by eyestrain, unless the history clearly suggests that it is only associated with the use of the eyes.

Bashed face

Traditionally faciomaxillary injuries are classified as to whether they primarily affect the upper (skull), middle or lower (mandibular) thirds of the head (*Figure 5.11*). Within each third, various bones or combination of bones, may be fractured in different ways though none are obviously more common than others. The two commonest sites are the nasal and skull (upper third) bones and these are dealt with elsewhere (pages 86 and 168). Otherwise the commonest area to be bashed is the middle third of the face and the most severe injuries are caused in road traffic accidents where the car occupant, who is not wearing a seat belt, is thrown against the dashboard or windscreen. Sports injuries (from a ball, racket, stick, opponent's head or fist) are more common but thankfully usually less serious.

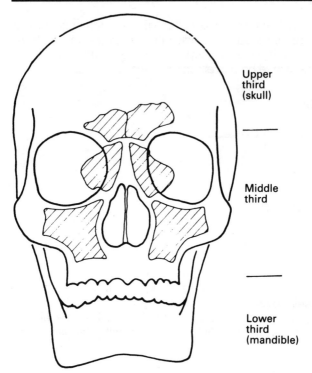

Upper
third
(skull)

Middle
third

Lower
third
(mandible)

Figure 5.11   General classification of faciomaxillary injuries

In determining whether there actually is a facial fracture, as opposed to just soft tissue swelling and bruising, clinical examination is extremely useful. When palpating to elicit local tenderness over a potential fracture site, knowledge of the usual sites of fracture is extremely useful. Intra-oral examination is also most important. The interrelationship of the teeth or the jaw in the dentulous patient should be assessed as this is often the easiest way to detect a displaced fracture in this area. Palpation of the intra-oral structures to detect local tenderness is also extremely important. Enquiries about diplopia and examination of eye movement to detect muscle entrapment will usually detect any serious involvement of the orbit by a fracture. Finally, as the infra-orbital nerve is commonly injured by a fracture, it is important to examine the area of the face it supplies (*Figure 5.12*) and compare the patient's sensation of touch to a piece of cotton wool over this area with that on the non-injured side.

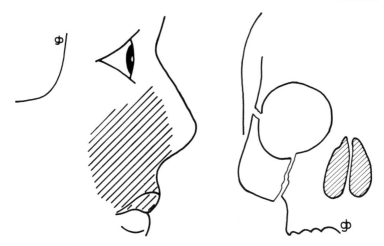

Figure 5.12   Sensory area supplied
by infra-orbital nerve

Figure 5.13   Zygomatic fractures

Radiology determines more precisely the position of a fracture and hence is of considerable benefit in deciding the management. Repeat radiological examination to ensure that the fracture has been satisfactorily reduced is, of course, essential. The following are the signs of the commoner fractures not dealt with elsewhere, along with an indication of how they are most frequently managed.

Zygomatic fracture (*Figure 5.13*)

Signs

1. Orbital margin step.
2. Flattened cheek, especially when viewed from above.
3. Possible asymmetry of eyes with resultant diplopia.
4. Possible infra-orbital nerve paraesthesia.

Management

Manipulative reduction via an incision at the hairline in front of the ear. After reduction, if it is unstable, wiring or maxillary antral packing is used.

Blow out orbital fracture (*Figure 5.14*)

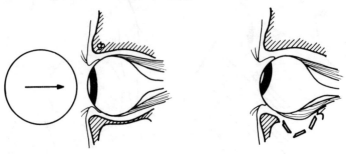

Figure 5.14   Blow out fracture of orbital floor

Signs

Limited eye movement due to trapping of orbital muscles by the fragmented bone.

Management

Open reduction via the orbit or maxillary antrum.

Le Fort fractures (*Figure 5.15*)

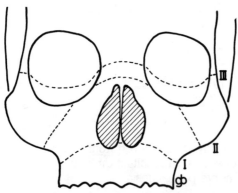

Figure 5.15   Sites for the Le Fort fracture of the middle third

Signs

1. Flattened face often with potentially fatal airway obstruction.
2. Non-alignment of upper and lower dentition or jaws.

Management

Manipulative reduction with either internal or external fixation and interdental splinting.

Mandibular fractures (*Figure 5.16*)

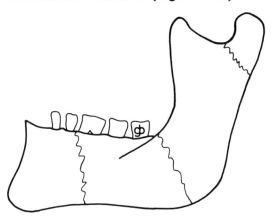

Figure 5.16   Common sites for mandibular fractures

Signs

1. Limited jaw movement due to reflex spasm.
2. Localized intra-oral tenderness.
3. Possible non-alignment of upper and lower dentition.

Management

Interdental splinting.

■ Conclusions

- Displaced fractures of the middle third of face can usually be diagnosed by clinical examination, especially by palpation.
- Intra-oral examination is especially important.

- Orbital involvement with diplopia and infra-orbital nerve paraesthesia are relatively common.
- Management varies depending on the stability of the reduced fragments. If unstable, wiring or splinting with a halo or packing is necessary.

Otolaryngological aspects of head injury

To many, the initial reaction must be 'What on earth have head injuries to do with ENT?' Unfortunately, this reaction reflects the present attitude regarding the role of an ENT surgeon in the management of head injuries and is to the detriment of both the patient and the medical profession. The initial aim of those managing head injuries is, naturally, to maintain the airway and ensure that the circulating blood volume is adequate. Once this has been done the general extent of injuries to the body is assessed as well as the extent and degree of damage to the head. It is to assess the latter that the ENT surgeon can be of considerable benefit, because it is he who can examine most competently the orifices of the skull (ear, nose, mouth) as well as assess the function of the cranial nerves, which are commonly injured as they pass through the skull foramina. This clinical examination is crucial for diagnosis as ancillary investigations, particularly radiology, do not define function.

That the ENT surgeon merits a place in the team managing acute head injuries should be without dispute and is strongly supported by the considerations below. His place is just as important in the long-term management, especially in the evaluation of vertigo and hearing loss which frequently occur.

The term 'head injury' covers a range of injuries to the soft tissues of the head, the skull and its contents but, contrary to what might be expected, the degree of intracranial damage is not directly proportional to the degree of skull damage. Thus, a patient can be deeply unconscious without any skull fracture and alternatively, fully alert with an extensive fracture. The diagnosis and management of a patient with a head injury is thus first of the concussive effects of head injury, secondly of any fracture or its complications.

Head injury without fracture

Sudden movement of the intracranial contents within the skull cavity occasioned by a head injury, can stretch the cranial nerve fibres. Once a cranial nerve fibre has been stretched its recovery is slow and can be the cause of long-term dysfunction. Thus, the olfactory nerve is often stretched or torn at the cribriform plate and, although loss of smell at the time of injury is not often noticed because of the more dominant nature of the other complaints, it is often complained of later. The other cranial nerve that can be damaged is the VIII nerve as it leaves the brain stem to run through the internal auditory canal to innervate the cochlea and the vestibular labyrinth. A considerable proportion of individuals with a severe head injury, without a skull fracture, have vertigo, tinnitus or loss of hearing which can be attributed to direct damage to the VIII nerve and the end organs of hearing and balance or to a whiplash injury to the cervical spine. The assessment of such patients is often difficult because of additional emotional problems and pending legal action for compensation. Complaints of loss of balance and hearing are most often real and should be considered seriously. Unfortunately, there is little that can be done at the time of injury to aid neural recovery and symptomatic measures are all that can be offered.

Head injury with skull fracture

Skull fractures can be either depressed or linear. Both can cause pressure symptoms by being associated with intracranial bleeding but linear fractures can, by extending some distance from the site of injury, involve the cranial nerves as they pass through the skull foramina. Fractures can involve either singly or in combination the temporal, parietal, frontal and occipital bones.

Temporal and parietal bone fractures

The temporal bone contains the ossicular chain and the end organs of hearing and balance supplied from the brain stem by the VIII cranial nerve. In addition, the temporal bone is closely integrated with the parietal bone, so that blows to the side of the head, and hence to the parietal bone, frequently involve the temporal bone. If alert enough to respond, a patient with an injury to the temporal or parietal bone may complain of dullness of hearing, of disturbance of balance, of tinnitus or of any combination.

The diagnosis of a temporal bone fracture is clinical rather than radiological. In assessing whether there is a temporal or parietal bone injury the area around the ear is palpated for tenderness and swelling. The external ear and the external auditory canal are then examined. If blood is found in the canal, and if alternative sources for this, such as lacerations, can be excluded, this is considered diagnostic of a middle cranial fossa fracture involving the temporal bone. The blood in the ear has come via a traumatic perforation of the tympanic membrane (which often cannot be seen because of the blood) from a fracture extending from the middle cranial fossa to the middle ear. A cerebrospinal fluid leak is not usually evident initially because of the blood, but it should be assumed to be likely.

If there is no blood in the external auditory canal, there may be blood in the middle ear (haemotympanum), evident by a blue discoloration of the tympanic membrane. This alone will give a mild conductive hearing impairment which resolves spontaneously within about four weeks. In addition, the ossicular chain may be disrupted, most often by the incus being dislocated. This results in a more severe hearing impairment than a haemotympanum, and if spontaneous resolution does not occur, surgical correction is required. On the other hand if the external auditory canal and the tympanic membrane are normal, a temporal bone injury cannot be excluded. In all cases a hearing assessment must be performed as soon as the patient is cooperative, and the results should be confirmed by pure tone audiometry. A sensorineural hearing impairment especially of the high frequencies, is all too common.

If a fracture is suspected it is normal to prescribe prophylactic antibiotics such as penicillin and sulphadimidine to prevent intracranial infection from bacteria gaining access via the fracture line. Otherwise the management is expectant. In those with a sensorineural hearing impairment there may be some return of hearing although this may take many months because of the slow rate of neural regeneration. In those with disequilibrium the symptoms should also settle but again this may take many months.

On the other hand if a sensorineural hearing impairment or vertigo is becoming progressively worse, surgical exploration and packing off of the fracture line to prevent the cerebrospinal fluid leak is warranted to halt and hopefully reverse the trend.

A facial nerve palsy is a relatively uncommon complication of a temporal bone fracture but if complete and occurring immediately following the injury, warrants surgical exploration of the ear to reappose the damaged ends of the nerve.

Frontal bone fracture

The frontal sinuses are within, and the olfactory nerves pass through, the frontal bones. Stretching or tearing of the olfactory nerve can occur without a frontal bone fracture, but is more frequent when there is one. With a fracture a tract is often opened from the subarachnoid space to the nose, resulting in a leak of bloody cerebrospinal fluid. This can pass unnoticed as the volume of the leak may not be large and follows the natural route of drainage from the nose via the nasopharynx to the pharynx. Sometimes, however, the patient may notice a salty taste in the mouth. It is usually only when there are copious amounts of cerebrospinal fluid that it overflows via the anterior nares and becomes clinically evident. Anterior and posterior rhinoscopy should, therefore, be performed in any patient in whom a frontal bone fracture is suspected. Any watery or bloody fluid which is present is collected for analysis. The distinction of cerebrospinal fluid from a mucoid nasal discharge is most easily done by quantitative assessment of glucose, the level of this being higher in cerebrospinal fluid than in mucus. Dextrostix are often used to do this but their use is invalidated by the presence of blood, quantitative biochemical analysis then being mandatory.

Lateral radiology of the skull can on occasions delineate blood or cerebrospinal fluid levels within the frontal sinuses or intracranial air (pneumatocele) which has entered the skull via the fracture from the nose. Both of these radiological findings are considered diagnostic of a frontal bone fracture.

The management of frontal bone fracture, as of most skull fractures, is usually expectant. It is customary to prescribe prophylactic antibiotics with the aim of preventing meningitis from nasal organisms. Spontaneous closure of the cerebrospinal fluid leak is usual within ten days but if prolonged thereafter may necessitate obliteration of the frontal sinus or neurosurgical closure of the dural tear.

Occipital bone fractures

As no structures are in or pass through the occipital bone, the only complications of its fracture are intracranial. This is, therefore, the only skull bone fracture where an ENT examination does not particularly aid in diagnosis.

■ Conclusions

- A severe head injury without a skull fracture is often complicated by hearing and vestibular disorders.
- Haemotympanum or blood (and cerebrospinal fluid) in the external auditory canal is diagnostic of a middle cranial fossa fracture involving the temporal bone.
- These individuals almost invariably have a hearing loss and balance problems which may merit surgical intervention.
- A facial palsy occurring immediately following a head injury is also diagnostic of a temporal bone fracture and may merit surgical exploration.
- Loss of smell or a watery nasal discharge following a head injury suggests a frontal bone fracture.

Something stuck

Any ENT or casualty surgeon could, if he wished, build up a highly individual collection of assorted objects which he has removed from the ear, nose or throat. The majority of these he would have removed from children and, in some, it will have been a chance finding when examining the patient for a cause of otorrhoea or rhinorrhoea.

The first attempt at removal of a foreign body is always the best. Good lighting, appropriate instruments and adequate head holding, especially of children, are, therefore, essential. The more attempts at removal there are, the more impacted the object may become, making removal under a general anaesthetic imperative.

Something in the ear

Pencil rubbers, beads, stones, cotton wool and other objects are often poked into the external auditory canal and lost. There need not necessarily be symptoms but otorrhoea (discharging ear) is often found to be due to a piece of cotton wool lost during cleaning with a cotton bud.

All objects are best removed by syringing, and this includes insects, which will be drowned. There is usually a gap between the posterosuperior canal wall and the object. The water should, therefore, be aimed at the posterior canal wall in order to bypass the object and force it out with the water after being reflected from the tympanic membrane. The ear must always be examined after the object has been removed as the initial reason for poking the ear may well be underlying pathology. The other ear must also be inspected, as it often contains another object.

Something in the nose

A foreign body in the nose often remains symptomless until there is such a foul stench (ozoena) due to superimposed infection that the parents think there must be something wrong with either the teeth or the tonsils.

Removal is achieved with the child sitting on or between the knees of a parent or nurse, with the head held upright and steady by hands placed over the ears. The foreign body usually lies on the nasal floor, lodged between the inferior turbinate and the septum. A curved Eustachian catheter can, therefore, be inserted over the object, which is then extracted, against the nasal floor (*Figure 5.17*).

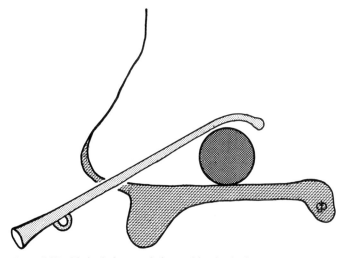

Figure 5.17   Method of removal of a nasal foreign body

Something in the throat

Sharp objects such as fish bones can stick anywhere in the mouth and pharynx but the areas of predilection are the tonsils, the base of the tongue, and the oropharynx. In the mouth and pharynx, as opposed to the oesophagus, patient localization of the object is reasonably accurate. Unfortunately, however, it is often difficult for the patient to differentiate between an object that remains lodged and one that has passed on. In the latter instance symptoms persist, presumably due to mild mucosa trauma. Impacted fish bones are not a danger to life, but should be removed because they are uncomfortable.

Solid objects do not usually stick until they reach the oesophagus, where there are three points that are relatively narrower. The first and usual point in children is at the oesophageal inlet in the postcricoid region. The second and third sites, especially in adults, are at the arch of the aorta and the cardio-oesophageal junction where there is often associated pathology (spasm, fibrosis, stricture or neoplasm). In the elderly it is surprising what is actually swallowed and gets stuck, lumps of meat and whole segments of orange being relatively common. This is because if the elderly wear any dentures at all they often only wear the upper ones which makes it difficult for them to chew.

Impacted oesophageal objects usually present as acute dysphagia because of the combined effect of obstruction and secondary spasm.

In order to identify the site of the foreign body a forehead light is essential, leaving both hands free to use the instruments. It is often better to spray the pharynx with a local anaesthetic (4 per cent lignocaine) early rather than late so that the patient's cooperation is retained. With the use of laryngeal mirrors and spatulae or tongue depressors, it should be possible to identify all objects lodged in the mouth and pharynx and remove them with angled forceps. If a foreign body cannot be identified, lateral X-rays of the neck can be helpful in localizing a radio-opaque object, fish bones sometimes coming into this category. The presence of a foreign body in the oesophagus can be suspected on mirror examination by pooling of saliva at the oesophageal inlet. Anteroposterior radiological views of the chest can be helpful in the localization of opaque objects in the oesophagus but if negative, and symptoms are present, a foreign body must be assumed.

The management of solid objects in the oesophagus varies. Operative removal requires a general anaesthetic and the passing of a rigid oesophagoscope, both of which have a definite morbidity and mortality. It is not an uncommon experience to find that on passing the scope the object has spontaneously passed on in the time lapse between admission and endoscopy. The majority of oesophageal foreign bodies will do little harm so a period of observation is not dangerous but endoscopy is always performed for sharp objects because of the fear and dangers of perforation.

Endoscopy also tends to be performed earlier with large objects and in children where the hold up is at the cricopharyngeal sphincter. Otherwise, the policy is to wait and only intervene if spontaneous passage has not occurred within 24 hours. In adults it is wise to exclude any pathology, especially at the gastro-oesophageal junction, so if endoscopy is not carried out because the object has spontaneously passed on, a barium swallow should be subsequently performed.

■ Conclusions

- The first attempt at removal of any foreign body is always the best.
- Foreign bodies in the ear are best removed by syringing.
- Foreign bodies in the nose are best removed by a curved probe.
- Foreign bodies in the mouth and pharynx are best removed with angled forceps.
- Foreign bodies in the oesophagus can be left to see if they pass on spontaneously, unless they are sharp and likely to perforate the wall. Surgical removal is via a rigid oesophagoscope.

Appendix: When to refer

Referral patterns to otorhinolaryngologists vary from country to country and within a country from area to area depending on the experience and facilities of the referrer and of the specialist. However, in the British context it is possible to lay down some general guidelines as to who should be referred and with what degree of urgency.

Mandatory referral within 24 hours

Uncontrollable epistaxis	To prevent death.
Stridor	To prevent death by intubation, humidification, steroid and antibiotic administration, removal of foreign body or treatment of acute epiglottitis and tumours
Nasal and faciomaxillary trauma	For consideration of manipulation or fixation.
Facial palsy	If there is any question of otological pathology or head injury.
Sudden hearing loss	All cases in which wax or otitis media with effusion is not the cause; for assessment, monitoring and perhaps early treatment.

Mandatory referral as soon as possible

Obvious head and neck
tumours

Non-inflammatory neck lumps	To exclude a head and neck primary neoplasm.
Unilateral nasal polyps	To exclude a neoplasm.
Upper alimentary dysphagia	To exclude an oral or pharyngeal neoplasm.
Unilateral hearing impairment	To exclude a nasopharyngeal neoplasm and acoustic neuroma.

Recommended referral for investigation and management

Hearing impairment that is disabling
Disabling vertigo
Disabling tinnitus
Active chronic otitis media

Conditions not usually requiring referral

Wax
Otitis externa
Transient acute otitis media
Transient otitis media with effusion
Transient sore throats
Allergic rhinitis
Chronic sinusitis

Index